AF327426

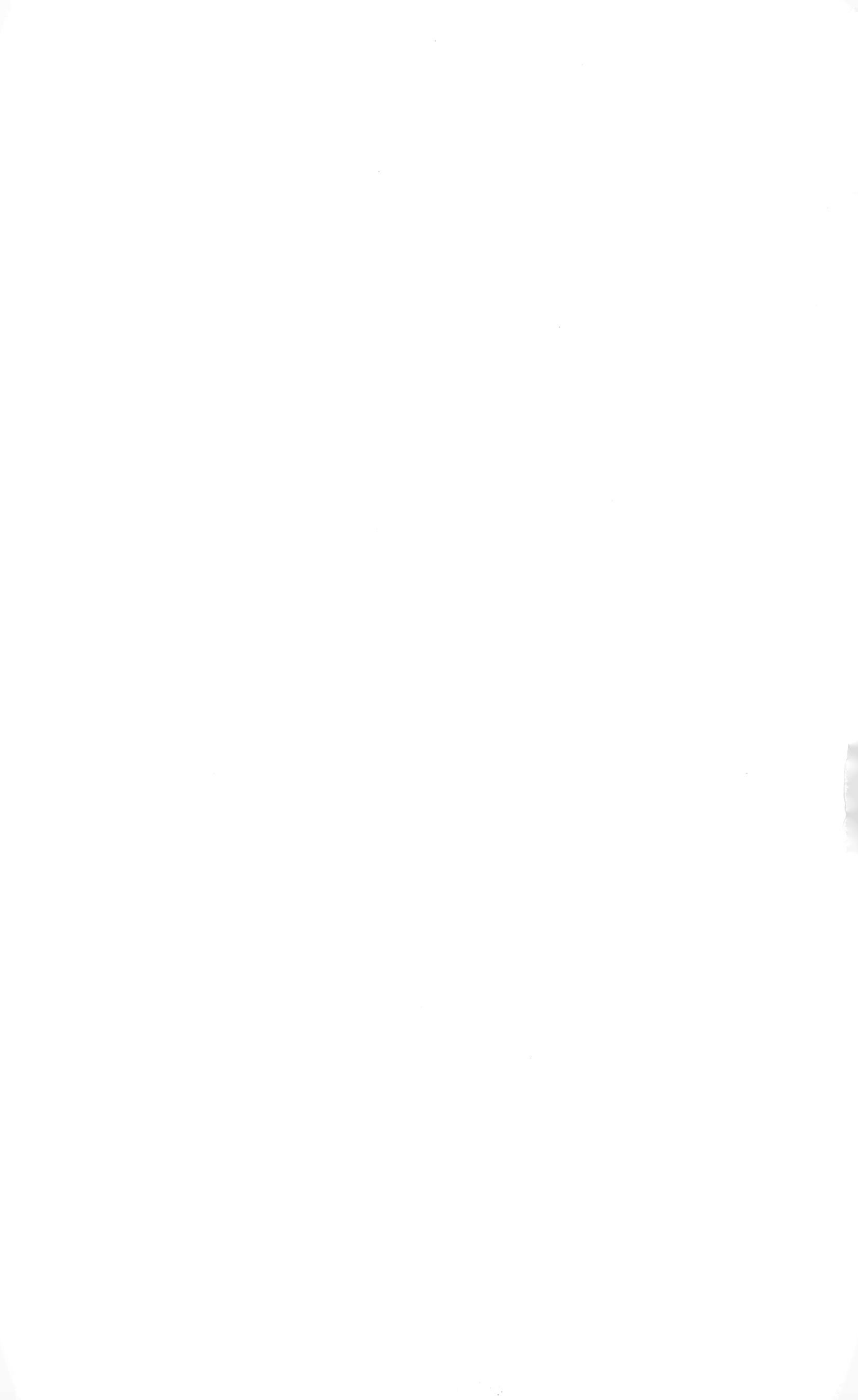

NEW TRENDS IN BODY MASS INDEX RESEARCH

HUMAN ANATOMY AND PHYSIOLOGY

Additional books in this series can be found on Nova's website
under the Series tab.

Additional E-books in this series can be found on Nova's website
under the E-books tab.

PHYSIOLOGY - LABORATORY AND CLINICAL RESEARCH

Additional books in this series can be found on Nova's website
under the Series tab.

Additional E-books in this series can be found on Nova's website
under the E-books tab.

HUMAN ANATOMY AND PHYSIOLOGY

NEW TRENDS IN BODY MASS INDEX RESEARCH

ALARD VERMEULEN
AND
EDME DE SMET
EDITORS

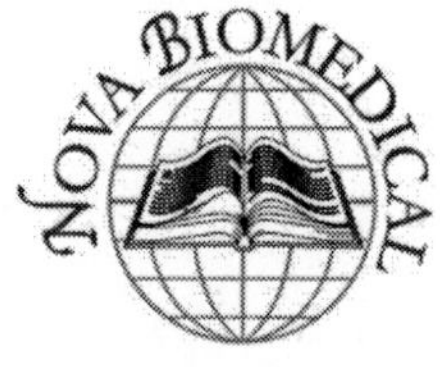

Nova Science Publishers, Inc.
New York

NOTICE TO THE READER

Additional color graphics may be available in the e-book version of this book.

Library of Congress Cataloging-in-Publication Data

New trends in body mass index research / editors, Alard Vermeulen and Edme De Smet.
p. cm.
Includes index.
ISBN 978-1-61942-430-2 (hardcover)
1. Obesity--Research. I. Vermeulen, Alard. II. De Smet, Edme.
RC628.N39 2011
616.3'98--dc23
2011047275

Published by Nova Science Publishers, Inc. † New York

CONTENTS

PREFACE

Body Mass Index (BMI) is the measure of the body weight relative to height that is associated with body fat and health risk. In this book, the authors present current research in the study of BMI including such topics as BMI and estrogen-dependent breast cancer in postmenopausal women; body mass index relating to psoriasis and age and sex variations in BMI.

Chapter 1 - Breast cancer is the female malignant neoplasia with the highest incidence in the industrialized world. Despite many undeniable therapeutic successes obtained, breast cancer still remains, however, a major health issue. In the last few years, thanks to aromatase inhibitors, the hormone therapy for estrogen-dependent breast cancer has evolved in terms of efficacy and tolerability; at the same time, it has enabled us to better define the role of estrogens in the etiopathogenesis of this tumor. Weight increase and obesity have been identified as the most important risk and prognostic factors for breast cancer in postmenopausal women. Several hypotheses have been proposed to explain the association of obesity with postmenopausal breast cancer. A more recent hypothesis suggests that adipocytes and their autocrine (paracrine and endocrine actions) are at the centre of such an etiopathogenetic mechanism. A better understanding of the main mechanisms that link together menopause, body-weight increase and hormone-dependent breast cancer is paramount to enable the identification of key molecules involved in the development of breast carcinoma and suggest new therapeutic options.

The present review will discuss important findings on the therapeutic aspects of adipose tissue and adipokines as a target for treatment of hormone-dependent breast cancer.

Chapter 2 - Overweight and obesity are related with several chronic diseases, such as cardiovascular disease (CVD), and its prevalence is rapidly increasing worldwide. Body mass index (BMI) has been used as a good tool to measure obesity; however, some authors claim that it may provide surrogate information about CVD risk. Nonetheless, the value of the associations between the different anthropometric measures that could be used with CVD risk and with its risk factors are similar, providing, therefore, comparable information.

Psoriasis is a chronic inflammatory skin disease that affects about 2-3% of the population. There are several risk factors associated with psoriasis appearance, progression and severity, namely smoking, alcohol consumption, depression, repeated physical traumas and major stressful events. Moreover, psoriasis has been associated with overweight and obesity. Indeed, the prevalence of obesity in psoriatic patients seems to be higher than that observed in the general population. An average BMI of 28 to 30 kg/m^2 has been reported for psoriatic patients.

The relationship between a high BMI and psoriasis is not completely understood. Some studies refer that overweight or obesity, appear after the onset of psoriasis, while others suggest that obesity precedes and may represent a risk factor for psoriasis. The pro-inflammatory state of obesity, may, in part, explain its association with psoriasis. The release of pro-inflammatory cytokines and the altered secretion of adipokines may contribute to the pathologic changes observed in psoriasis.

The prevalence of high BMI in psoriatic patients seems to be strongly associated with an increased risk for CVD. Besides overweight/obesity, psoriasis associates with several others risk factors for CVD that might explain the prevalence of CVD events in these patients.

A high BMI may influence the therapeutic approach to psoriasis and the clinical response to treatment. Indeed, an increased BMI appears to affect negatively the initial response to treatments. In opposition, a normal or a reduction of BMI may favor/complement the treatment of psoriatic patients.

In summary, a complex relationship between BMI, psoriasis, psoriasis treatment and psoriasis morbidity and mortality exists, suggesting the need for a multidisciplinary approach in the management of patients with psoriasis. Psoriatic patients should be surveyed for both dermatological and metabolic aspects, in order to guide for the best therapy, and to monitor patients during therapy and during the inactive phase of the disease.

Chapter 3 - The body mass index (BMI) is an indicator of body composition (BC) and adiposity in particular. This status is the result of good correlations with indirect two- and three-component models predicting adiposity. The BMI has become the most widely used measure to diagnose obesity and yet no accepted ranges of fat percentage exist. Although being overweight or obese is strongly associated to excess mortality in large cohorts, the accuracy of BMI in detecting excess body adiposity in individuals is largely unknown. Moreover its direct relationship with anatomical tissues in general and subcutaneous, intra-peritoneal and intra-muscular adiposity in particular is not established. Concurrently emerging evidence indicates that health-related assessment of BC in the elderly is more appropriate if muscle mass and adiposity are considered jointly, instead of separately. However it remains unclear how BMI (weight/height^2) and/or waist circumference (WC) relate to body tissue distribution in the elderly. Therefore the relationship of BMI and WC with body tissue masses, with muscle/adipose tissue mass ratios and with trunk adipose tissue distribution was explored by direct cadaver dissection. For this purpose post-mortem whole BC and segmental adipose tissue composition of twenty-nine Belgian elderly persons (17 females and 12 males, aged 78.1±6.9 years) was determined at the anatomical tissue-system level: i.e. skin, muscle, adipose tissue, viscera and bones. Results indicate that BMI and WC are significantly related to adipose and non-adipose tissue masses in both sexes. Whole body muscle mass, and whole body and segmental adipose tissue masses correlated better with BMI (r-values between 0.61 and 0.90) than with WC (r-values between 0.49 and 0.83). BMI was also significantly and inversely related with various muscle/adipose tissue ratios in both sexes (r-values between -0.54 and -0.68), and was positively related with trunk adipose tissue distribution (i.e. ratio of internal/total body adipose tissue and ratio of internal/subcutaneous trunk adipose tissue) in elderly females (r-values between 0.50 and 0.54), but not in males. Although BMI and WC are significantly related with muscle/adipose tissue mass ratios in elderly subjects, persons with similar tissue mass proportions do not necessarily fit within the same BMI or WC risk-category. The use of BMI and/or WC for the comparison of individual BC is therefore limited, particularly in the intermediate ranges. Since individual body tissue distribution varies considerably future research should focus on adjusting BMI and WC, or on developing more valid anthropometric parameters for clinical decision making in elderly persons.

Chapter 4 - This chapter was a cross-sectional one, undertaken to determine the prevalence of undernutrition using body mass index among 18 years and above Santali adults of Purulia District, West Bengal, India. A total of 791 (345 males and 446 females) adult from Santal habitat villages were measured. Commonly used indicators i.e., weight, height and BMI, are used to evaluate nutritional status. Significant ge-group difference both in males (F =

16.164, p < 0.001) and females (F = 8.213, p < 0.001) were recorded. Significant sex differences in mean BMI were observed in age range 18-39 years (t = 8.243, p < 0.001), age range 40-55 years (t = 2.899, p < 0.05) and age range > 55 years as (t = 2.242, p < 0.05). The females were highly energy deficient than their male counterpart; females have CED (Gd-III = 13.7, Gd-II = 16.1, Gd-I = 30.9) then males (Gd-III = 6.7, Gd-II = 6.4, Gd-I = 19.4). There was a highly significant difference between sexes in CED prevalence (x^2= 64.977; df = 4; p < 0.001). BMI was highly negatively significantly correlated with age and age^2. Sex had significant (F= 71.394, p< 0.001) effect on BMI. Even after controlling for age, sex explained 8.1% of variation in BMI. Santal adults of Purulia, India are in very critical situation for all age groups and the women and oldest among them were experiencing the most critical situation with respect to their health and nutritional status.

Chapter 5 - Information on the body size and distribution of body fat in circumpolar populations is of particular interest when examining the validity of simple methods of estimating the overall body fat content; use of the body mass index (BMI) is complicated by the atypical body build of the traditional Inuit and by the manner in which this historic phenotype has changed with acculturation to the lifestyle of industrialized society in recent years. Comparison of body mass index data with other measures of body fat content show that the former can give a misleading impression of obesity in populations with a short stature and/or a muscular body build. Over the past four de cades, the "natural experiment" of acculturation to southern Canadian patterns of diet and physical activity has led to rapid changes of physique among arctic populations, including a deterioration of physical fitness and a substantial increase of average body fat content. Skinfold readings suggest a substantial accumulation of body fat, but because of a reduction in lean tissue, this is not always reflected in the BMI. The replacement of hunting by the consumption of store-purchased food and the adoption of a sedentary lifestyle present nutritional and environmental challenges to many circumpolar populations, but poor metabolic health is not an inevitable consequence of adopting a "modern" lifestyle. As in urban, industrialized society, good health can be maintained through the deliberate incorporation of adequate physical activity into daily life.

Chapter 6 - Overweight/obesity (body mass index [BMI] of 25.0-29.9 and ≥ 30.0 kg/m^2 respectively) – now recognized as a major modifiable risk factor – is associated with higher risk of cardiovascular and non-cardiovascular morbidity and mortality, higher health care costs, and shorter life expectancy. Despite declines in prevalence of other key major cardiovascular disease

(CVD) risk factors such as hypercholesterolemia, high blood pressure, and cigarette smoking, prevalence of overweight and obesity has reached epidemic proportions and continues to rise with significant implications for the future health and well being of the aging population. While the short-term effects of BMI on quality of life (i.e., physical, mental and social well-being) are well established, the impact of BMI measured earlier in life on future health-related quality of life of men and women who survive to older ages has only recently been demonstrated. This chapter presents findings on the relation of BMI measured in middle age to health-related quality of life in older age (65 years and older), after an average follow-up of 31 years, among surviving participants from the Chicago Heart Association Detection Project in Industry (CHA). The CHA study is a prospective investigation of CVD risk factors. From late 1967 to early 1973, 39,522 men and women ages 18 and older, of varied ethnicities and socioeconomic levels, employed by 84 Chicago-area organizations, were screened. In 1996 and 2001, quality of life was assessed with widely used and standardized instruments, i.e., 12-item Health Status Questionnaire (HSQ-12), Medical Outcomes Trust 36-item Short-Form Health Survey (SF-36) performance of activities of daily living (ADL), and instrumental activities of daily living (IADL). Results demonstrate that higher BMI in middle age adversely impacts future health-related quality of life and physical functioning in older age. Conversely, for non-overweight persons (BMI 18.5-24.9 kg/m^2), preservation of health status and quality of life is evident, indicating that increasing life expectancy can be accompanied with disease-free and disability-free survival. With adverse BMI levels afflicting a large proportion of the US population and increasing numbers of people surviving to older ages, preventive measures are urgently required at younger ages to lessen future individual and societal burden of disease, health care costs, and also disability and impaired quality of life associated with excess weight.

In: New Trends in Body Mass Index Research   ISBN 978-1-61942-430-2
Editors: A. Vermeulen and E. De Smet   © 2012 Nova Science Publishers, Inc.

Chapter I

BODY MASS INDEX AND ESTROGEN-DEPENDENT BREAST CANCER IN POSTMENOPAUSAL WOMEN: PATHOGENETIC MECHANISMS AND NEW THERAPEUTIC PERSPECTIVES

Antonio Macciò[*,1] *and Clelia Madeddu*[2]

[1]Department of Obstetrics and Gynecology,Sirai Hospital, Carbonia, Italy
[2]Department of Medical Oncology, University of Cagliari, Cagliari, Italy

ABSTRACT

Breast cancer is the female malignant neoplasia with the highest incidence in the industrialized world. Despite many undeniable therapeutic successes obtained, breast cancer still remains, however, a major health issue. In the last few years, thanks to aromatase inhibitors, the hormone therapy for estrogen-dependent breast cancer has evolved in terms of efficacy and tolerability; at the same time, it has enabled us to better define the role of estrogens in the etiopathogenesis of this tumor. Weight increase and obesity have been identified as the most important risk and prognostic factors for breast cancer in postmenopausal women. Several hypotheses have been proposed to explain the association of obesity with postmenopausal breast cancer. A more recent hypothesis suggests that adipocytes and their autocrine (paracrine and endocrine actions) are at the centre of such an etiopathogenetic mechanism. A better understanding of the main mechanisms that link together menopause, body-weight increase and hormone-dependent breast cancer is paramount to enable the identification of key molecules involved in the development of breast carcinoma and suggest new therapeutic options.

The present review will discuss important findings on the therapeutic aspects of adipose tissue and adipokines as a target for treatment of hormone-dependent breast cancer.

INTRODUCTION

Breast cancer is the female gender malignant neoplasia with the highest incidence in the industrialized world. Despite many undeniable therapeutic successes obtained mainly thanks to early diagnosis, breast cancer however still remains a major health issue. About 60% of breast carcinomas are hormone- dependent. Therefore, a specific antagonist to the estrogen action or its deprivation must be considered as the most rational therapeutic approach for the prevention and treatment of hormone-dependent breast cancer.

In the last few years, thanks to the aromatase inhibitors, the hormone therapy for estrogen-dependent postmenopausal breast cancer has evolved in terms of efficacy and tolerability, and at the same time has enabled to better define the role of estrogens in the etiopathogenesis and evolution of this tumor. The hormonal changes in postmenopause, ascribable to a specific physical and metabolic remodelling, not only represent a greater risk for breast cancer, but are also to be considered indispensable for a more effective therapy (1).

Weight increase and obesity, subsequent to the menopause, have been identified as the most important risk and prognostic factors for breast cancer in postmenopausal women (Figure 1). A statistically significant increased risk (78% to 91%) of recurrence, and increased risk (36% to 56%) of death in women with breast cancer was associated with overweight and obesity (2).

According to this evidence, several hypotheses have been proposed to explain the association of obesity with postmenopausal breast cancer. The main one is that circulating estrogen levels from peripheral aromatization of androgens in obese postmenopausal women are higher than in slim postmenopausal women. A second hypothesis is that obesity, being associated with metabolic syndrome, results in increasingly circulating levels of insulin and insulin-like growth factor (IGF), which, by acting as mitogens for epithelial breast cells, stimulate their growth and neoplastic degeneration. A more recent hypothesis suggests that adipocytes and their autocrine, paracrine and endocrine actions are at the centre of such an etiopathogenetic mechanism (3). Adipocytes, once considered solely as energy depot cells, are actually recognized as active endocrine cells that secrete cytokines, polipeptides and hormone-like molecules. Indeed, the most likely hypothesis is that all these mechanisms may concur to explain the association which links together menopause, the subsequent body weight increase and hormone-dependent breast cancer.

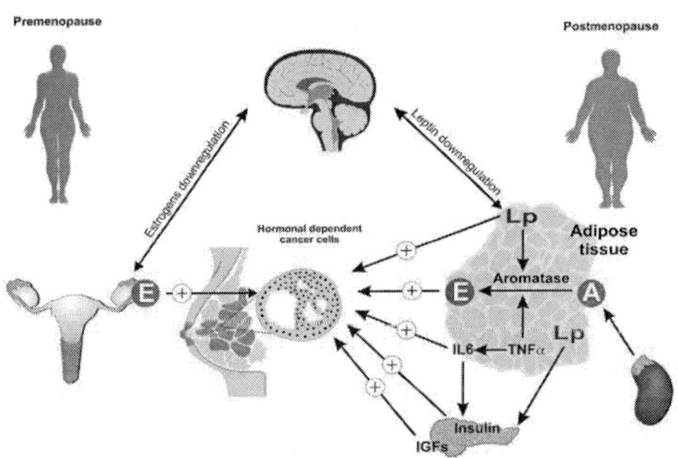

Figure 1. Different mechanisms of estrogen dependence for hormone-related breast cancer in pre- and postmenopausal women. In premenopausal women, the main site of synthesis of estrogen is the ovary. In postmenopausal women, adipose tissue is the main source of the circulating estrogens. Adipose tissue produces the enzymes aromatase; therefore, in obese women, there is an increased conversion of the androgens androstenedione and testosterone into the estrogens: oestrone and oestradiol, respectively, by aromatase. Moreover, obesity, being associated with metabolic syndrome, results in increasingly circulating levels of insulin and insulin-like growth factor, which, by acting as mitogens for epithelial breast cells, stimulate their neoplastic degeneration. Moreover, adipocytes produce several 'adipokines' such as leptin and inflammatory cytokines which can influence aromatase activity and estrogen-dependent cell proliferation. IGF, insulin growth factor; IL, interleukin; TNF-a, tumor necrosis factor-a; Lp, leptin; E, oestradiol; A, aromatase.

ESTROGENS AND MENOPAUSE

The most convincing, but indirect, evidence for a role of estrogen associated to obesity in postmenopausal breast cancer is that circulating levels of estrogen are strongly and linearly related to adiposity (4). Adipose tissue estrogens biosynthesis is catalized by the enzyme aromatase, a product of the CYP19 gene (5).

Beside the increased adipose mass, also its specific body distribution can contribute to breast tumorigenesis (6). Body fat distribution has been also correlated with breast cancer prognosis, with suggestions of increased breast cancer mortality risk with android body fat distribution defined as high waist-to-hip ratio, or a high suprailiac-to-thigh ratio (7).

Moreover, a central role is played by the adipose tissue that sustains and surrounds the breast glandular tissue and includes a mix of mature adipocytes, indifferentiated fibroblasts and macrophages. Variations in fibroblasts distribution may also regulate the local breast synthesis of estrogen, thus influencing the tumor development (8). Indeed, local estrogen levels in breast tumors are as much as 10 times greater than in the circulation of postmenopausal woman. It is important to bear in mind that the fibroblasts, as for quantity, tallies with that of adipocytes, and that both components influence each other in their peculiar functional capacity. In fact, there are adipose tissue specific promoters of stromal cells aromatase, such as the promoter I.4, which in turn are regulated by macrophagic cytokines and glucocorticoids (9). Furthermore, it seems that the increased aromatase expression in the adipose tissue of breast bearing carcinoma derives also from the activation of promoters II e 1.3, which are regulated by unknown factors presumably secreted by malignant epithelial cells: among these prostaglandin (PG) E2 seems to be a likely candidate (10).

There may be, however, an alternative mode of action for estrogens, which can be determined in this scenario. The dense layer of fibroblasts that make up the capsule surrounding premalignant or cancerous breast lesions may have high levels of aromatase activity thus enhancing estrogens biosynthesis. As a result, the histological composition of breast tissue may favour the estrogen-dependent growth and progression of breast cancer cells in a paracrine manner, in which the steroid spreads from its site of synthesis to interact with the ERs on nearby cancer cells. Moreover, some breast cancers have themselves aromatase activity, and in the presence of ER+ breast cancer cells are able to stimulate tumor growth by an autocrine mechanism (11).

WEIGHT INCREASE, INSULIN-RESISTANCE AND RISK OF BREAST CANCER

It has been widely demonstrated that body mass index (BMI) increase in postmenopausal women is not only associated with hyperestrogenism, but also with hyperinsulinemia and insulin-resistant type-2 diabetes which in turn are associated with a slight increase in the risk of hormone-dependent breast cancer (12).

Several hypothesis have been proposed to explain the association of obesity, related hyperestrogenism and hyperinsulinemia with postmenopausal breast cancer. The accumulation of visceral adipose tissue has been associated with insulin-resistance and dyslipidemia, and, therefore, the involvement of adipose tissue in the pathogenesis of breast cancer is consistent with the identification of type-2 diabetes and metabolic syndrome as risk factors for this tumor. In metabolic syndrome, tissues are not able to absorb, store and metabolize glucose efficiently. Therefore, to prevent elevated glucose concentrations in the blood, the pancreas secrete increasing amounts of insulin in both the fed and fasted states (13). In turn, insulin increases proliferation of ER+, but not ER-, breast cancer cell lines (14). Indeed, estrogens and insulin may cooperate through their differential regulation of c-Myc and cyclin D1 to promote cell-cycle progression (15) (Figure 2).

Hyperinsulinemia can also affect indirectly tumorigenesis by contributing to synthesis and activity of insulin-growth factor (IGF)-I and II, which have been increasingly recognized as critical to breast cancer. IGFs can act in an endocrine, paracrine or autocrine fashion to regulate cell growth, survival and differentiation and can synergize with other growth factors to enhance their mitogenic effect (16). Analysis of genetic polymorphism showed a significant correlation between the expression of specific insuline-related genes and increased risk of breast cancer in postmenopausal women exposed to estrogens. Approximately one-half of primary breast cancers overexpress the IGF-I receptor (IGF-IR), suggesting that these carcinomas have enhanced responses to the mitogenic and antiapoptotic effects of IGF-I (17). Conversely, the inactivation of IGF-IR results in reduced mammary tumor growth and metastasis *in vivo* (18). Binding of IGF-I to the specific receptor leads to its dimerization, activation of its tyrosine kinase activity and phosphorylation of key substrates which recruit different SH2-containing proteins and activate various intracellular pathways, including phosphatidylinositol 3-kinase (PI 3-kinase) and mitogen-activated protein kinase (MAPK) signaling cascade

(Figure 2). Both the PI 3-kinase and MAPK pathways are important for IGF-I-stimulated proliferation of MCF-7 human breast cancer cells and their inhibition abrogate IGFs' mitogenic effects (16).

Moreover, insuline and IGFs can activate ER transcriptional activity in breast cancer cell lines, even in the absence of estrogens. The estradiol in the presence of IGF-I is able to induce the trascriptional activation of ER to levels higher than observed with the ligand alone, while loss of ER leads to a

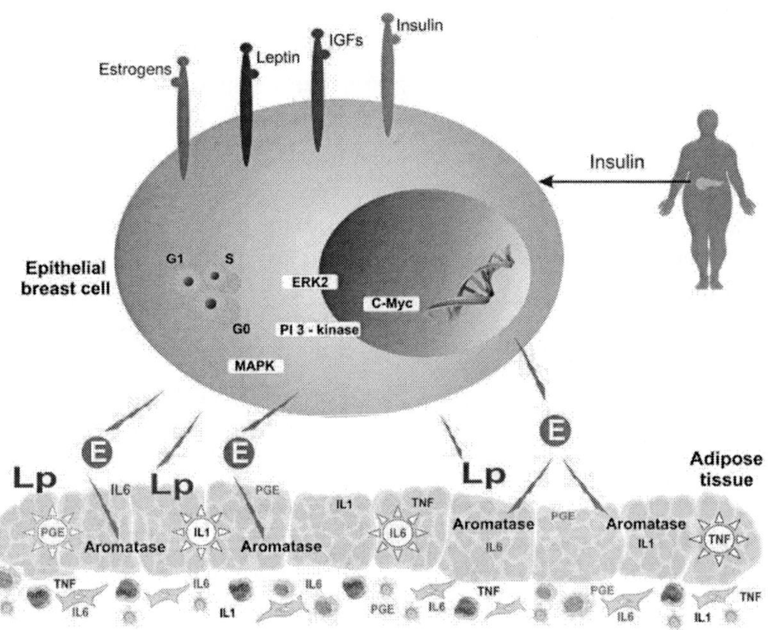

Figure 2. Molecular mechanisms regulating breast cancer cell proliferation by paracrine and endocrine adipose tissue-derived factors. In obesity, insulin and IGF-I serum levels are elevated and interact with estrogen cellular pathways to synergistically induce the mitogenic response in breast epithelial cells. Moreover, adipocytes act as both a peripheral site of estrogen aromatization and a paracrine source of multiple adipokines and inflammatory mediators. Among adipokines, leptin is able to influence different second intracellular messengers involved in the breast cancer cell proliferation and survival such as STAT3, transcription AP-1, ERK2 and MAPK. All these factors act to support and promote tumor cell proliferation and progression. AP-1, activator protein 1; E, oestradiol; ERK2, extracellular signal regulated kinase-2; IGF, insulin growth factor; IL, interleukin; Lp, leptin; MAPK, mitogen-activated protein kinase; PGE, prostaglandin E; PI 3-kinase, phosphoinositide 3-kinase; TNF, tumor necrosis factor.

decrease in IGF-I signaling and mitogenic activity (19). Thus, the insulin-IGF-I pathway interacts with estrogens to synergistically induce the mitogenic response in breast epithelial cells.

Given that obese postmenopausal women have more estrogens, IGF-I and insulin than slim women, it is logical to conclude that the above described crosstalk between the IGF pathways and estrogen-mediated signalling may favour an increased risk of breast cancer to a greater extent in obese postmenopausal women (20).

It is to be underlined that, as adipose tissue mass increases circulating concentrations of insulin and IGF-I, blood levels of sex hormone-binding globulin (SHBG) begin to diminish (21). Since SHBG binds estrogens with high affinity, its decrease results in an increased bioavailable fraction of circulating estradiol. Accordingly, in postmenopausal women blood levels of SHBG are inversely correlated with breast cancer risk (22). Additionally, SHBG may act directly on breast cancer cells to inhibit estradiol-induced proliferation. Thus, SHBG appears to be a regulator of estradiol action in breast cancer cells, acting as an anti-proliferative factor, loss of which in obese women could contribute to tumorigenesis (23).

ADIPOCYTES AND BREAST CANCER

It has been clearly shown that the adipose tissue is a complex and metabolically active endocrine organ. It contains, besides adipocytes, a connective matrix, nerve tissue, vascular and immune cells. Although the adipocytes synthesize and secrete several hormones, such as leptin and adiponectin, many proteins are produced by the nonadipocyte fraction of the adipose tissue, i.e. fibroblasts and macrophages that infiltrate the adipose cell mass: all these factors are known as "adipokines" (24).

Besides the storage and energy regulation function, the adipose tissue is equipped with the metabolic machinery which enables its communication with distant organs, including the central nervous system (CNS). The adipose tissue is thus an actual endocrine organ, fully involved in coordinating a number of biological processes, such as energy metabolism, neuroendocrine and immune functions. Indeed, adipokines including leptin, Tumor Necrosis Factor (TNF)-α, interleukin-6 (IL-6) and hepatocyte growth factors (HGF), apart from exerting their specific local biological effects, circulate in the plasma at concentrations positively correlated with BMI; one exception is adiponectin, which is inversely correlated with BMI (11).

Several in vitro and in vivo studies demonstrated that adypocytes can directly influence breast tumor growth. Microarray analysis revealed that MCF-7 breast cancer cells treated with adipocyte-conditioned media upregulated genes involved in invasion, proliferation, and metastasis, while simultaneously downregulating p18 and BARD1, a cell-cycle checkpoint inhibitor and tumor suppressor, respectively (25). *In vivo* tumors formed from SUM-159PT human breast adenocarcinoma cells co-injected with murine adipocytes grew to more than three times the size of tumors co-injected with murine fibroblast (26). *Viceversa*, the role of preadipocytes in tumor growth is controversal and, therefore, further studies are needed to elucidate their role in breast tumorigenesis.

Two adipokines, leptin and adiponectin, have been recently studied for their influence on the breast cancer risk and tumor biology. Their biological activities as their effects on breast neoplastic cells are largely in opposition to each other. A third adipokine, the HGF, can have a positive effect on tumor development as a result of its specific angiogenic properties and capacity to promote neoplastic invasion. Different roles are played by IL-6, TNF-α and resistin (11).

Leptin

Leptin, a product of the Ob gene, is a 16-kDa protein containing 167-amino acids with structural homology to cytokines. Leptin exerts its effects through binding to the leptin receptor (Ob-R), a member of the cytokine transmembrane receptor class I superfamily. Leptin is secreted by adipocytes proportionally to BMI as well as nutritional status and acts mainly upon the hypothalamus to regulate food intake and energy metabolism (27). It is also synthesised by preadipocytes, especially when these are stimulated in a paracrine way by the proinflammatory cytokines (TNF-α and IL-1β) secreted by the macrophages infiltrating the adipose tissue (28).

In addition to its effects on energy metabolism, leptin regulates some neuroendocrine systems. Other important endocrine actions of leptin include the regulation of the immune function, hematopoiesis, angiogenesis and bone development. Taking into account its numerous endocrine functions, leptin can be considered the prototype for all the adipose tissue-derived hormones.

The effects of leptin on energy homeostasis have been well demonstrated. Although leptin was initially considered an antiobesity hormone, its main role is that of signalling the availability of adequate energy reserves. Circulating leptin levels rapidly decline under caloric restriction and weight loss. This decline is associated to a number of adaptative physiological mechanisms such as the increase of appetite and reduction of resting energy expenditure. On the contrary, weight gain and the most common forms of obesity are characterized by high circulating leptin levels. Obesity is characterized by a condition of leptin-resistance whose mechanism may depend either from a defect in leptin signalling or transport across the blood-brain barrier. Indeed, mutations that lead to a lack of functional leptin or its receptor, although rare, result in extreme obesity in humans.

The discovery of leptin as a product of the adipose tissue has rapidly led to hypothesise a correlation between its circulating levels and breast cancer risk. Secretion of leptin seems to be associated not only with body weight regulation but also with sexual hormones production. Levels of estradiol, progesterone and leptin increase in the blood of breast cancer patients (29). Women with breast cancer have higher leptin plasma levels and mRNA expression in adipose tissue as compared to healthy subjects (30). Goodwin et al. (31) observed an association between high plasma leptin concentrations and high tumor stage, grade and negative steroid hormone receptor status, whilst there was no clear-cut relationship between serum leptin levels and disease outcome.

The mechanism through which leptin promotes breast tumor growth is complex. Recent studies have demonstrated that leptin is able to influence different second intracellular messengers involved in breast cancer cell proliferation and survival, such as signal transducers and activators of transcription 3 (STAT3), transcription activator protein 1 (AP-1), extracellular signal regulated kinase-2 (ERK2) and mitogen activated protein kinase (MAPK) (Figure 2). These mechanisms of signal transduction seem to be involved in the regulation of aromatase expression, estrogen synthesis and ER activation (32). In any case, leptin effects appear to be primarily mediated through ER action. There is evidence that leptin results in the direct activation of ER in MCF-7 breast cancer cells even in the absence of its natural ligand (33). Leptin also upregulates estradiol/ERα signaling in MCF-7 cells exposed to aromatizable androgen, and this signal is downregulated by the aromatase inhibitors.

Leptin gene expression occurs both in normal mammary tissue and solid tumors (34). However, overexpression of leptin as well as of its receptor, as determined by staining intensity, was observed in cancer cells but not in normal mammary epithelium. Interestingly, leptin and Ob-R tumoral overexpression are negative prognostic factors, associated with presence of distant metastasis and short survival (35).

Leptin interferes also with the insulin signalling, and plasma levels of leptin directly correlated with the degree of insulin-resistance in patients with type-2 diabetes (36), whose association with breast carcinoma is well known. At the same time, serum leptin levels are not significantly different between premenopausal breast cancer patients and healthy women (37). This result confirmed that leptin presumably does not influence mammary tumorigenesis in peri/premenopause but is a specific factor of postmenopause correlated with weight and hyperestrogenism. Indeed, it has been recently demonstrated that serum leptin levels significantly correlate with total body aromatasic activity in postmenopausal breast cancer patients (38).

Adiponectin

Adiponectin (ApN) is a 30 kDA polipeptide specifically secreted from adipocytes which circulates in serum in several different size isoforms. ApN acts through its two receptors, AdipoR1 and AdipoR2, which are expressed widely in various tissues, including breast tissue. Binding of ApN to its receptors activates AMP-activated protein kinase (AMPK) and peroxisome proliferator-activates receptor (PPAR)-γ metabolic pathways, leading to an increase in fatty acid oxidation, glucose uptake, and a decreased rate of gluconeogenesis, thus enhancing insulin sensitivity (39). The physiologic functions of ApN are mainly endocrine, but it exerts also paracrine actions, such as the inhibition of the leptin-induced production of TNF-α by macrophages (40).

ApN biosynthesis is inhibited by the increase of fat concentrations in adipocytes and therefore its circulating levels are lower in obese or overweight patients. Serum levels of ApN are inversely correlated with waist circumference and visceral fat, even more than with BMI. Low levels of ApN are associated with several metabolic diseases, such as obesity and insulin-resistance in type-2 diabetes, and inflammatory conditions (41). Conversely, ApN levels increase after weight reduction or treatment with insulin-sensitizing drugs, such as thiazolidinedione agonists of PPAR-γ (42).

Studies confirm a significant inverse correlation between serum ApN levels, breast cancer risk and poor-prognosis, independently from hormone receptor status (43). Little is known regarding the potential of ApN to directly influence the breast cancer cell growth, proliferation and differentiation. ApN inhibits the proliferation of several cell types and is a negative regulator of angiogenesis (44). It has been shown that ApN, binding to its receptors, activates the PPAR-γ pathway, which in turn induces the transcription of several genes involved in the regulation of cell proliferation and differentiation. Previous studies have demonstrated the importance of PPARs in the pathogenesis of breast cancer (45). A plausibile explanation of the association between ApN levels and breast carcinoma risk is that the reduction of ApN may result in a decreased activation of PPAR signaling and low nuclear levels of BRCA1 with subsequent damage to DNA repair mechanisms. Therefore, overweight subjects with low serum levels of ApN could also have an increased risk of developing tumors with an aggressive phenotype and enhanced neoangiogenesis.

Hepatocyte Growth Factor

The adipocytes and the stromal cells of the adipose tissue seem to be one of the main sources of HGF synthesis and therefore, it should be rightfully considered as an adipokine. Serum HGF levels positively correlate with BMI, and decrease following body weight loss (46). The HGF exerts several functions which influence the development and metastatisation of breast cancer. Stroma fibroblasts are the main source of HGF and their interaction with the breast epithelial cells is the basic requirement needed to enable HGF's oncogene, proangiogenetic and metastasing action. Serum HGF levels have been demonstrated to significantly correlate with high stage, ER-, degree of differentiation and presence of lymph node and distant metastases in patients with locally advanced breast cancer (47).

Tumor Necrosis Factor-A

TNFα was the first inflammatory cytokine to be identified as a product of adipocytes. Within the adipose tissue TNF-α is produced by adipocytes, stromavascular cells and macrophages and its expression is greater in the subcutaneous than in the visceral adipose tissue. Both in experimental models and in humans, adipose tissue expression of TNF-α increases with obesity and is positively correlated with the amount of adipose tissue and insulin-resistance (48). It is unknown the extent to which TNF-α produced by the adipose tissue is secreted in the circulation, even though a correlation between TNF-α levels and obesity indices has been reported (49).

TNF-α in the adipose tissue acts both in an autocrine and paracrine way to influence a range of processes, including apoptosis and synthesis of other cytokines and adipokines (50). Interestingly, recent studies have demonstrated that TNF-α regulates IL-6 synthesis and aromatase expression in the adipose tissue, thus stimulating estrogen production (51). Moreover, TNF-α induces IL-6 production via ERK1 activation in human MDA-MB-231 breast cancer cells (52). Moreover, it has been suggested that TNF-α plays a role in the development of insulin-resistance through the inhibition of the insulin receptor-signalling pathway (53). Thus, overweight subjects may have increased circulating TNF-α levels that could promote breast tumorigenesis through the induction of insulin-resistance and IL-6 and estrogens biosynthesis.

Interleukin-6 (IL-6)

IL-6 is an inflammatory cytokine involved in the immune response to cancer and plays an important role in tumor progression. IL-6 increases following menopause in healthy women (54), also released by adipocytes and, by acting both locally and in a systemic fashion, could disrupt the synthesis of estrogens. Polymorphisms in the IL6 gene promoter have been reported to be related to circulating levels of C-reactive protein (55), to be associated with different profiles of plasma IL-6 response to immunization (56).

Within the adipose tissue, IL-6 and its receptor are expressed by the adipocytes and the adipose tissue matrix. The expression and the secretion of IL-6 are 2-3 times greater in the visceral than in the subcutaneous adipose tissue. Both IL-6 plasma levels and its expression in the adipose tissue are high under obesity and insulin-resistance conditions. Moreover, circulating IL-6 levels are predictive of the development of type-2 diabetes and cardiovascular diseases (57).

Interestingly, IL-6 has several effects on energy homeostasis both peripherally and centrally. IL-6 peripherally inhibits lipogenesis and adiponectin secretion and centrally regulates the body energy homeostasis. It has been suggested that IL-6, together with leptin, could be responsible for conveying the information for the regulation of energy balance from the adipocytes to the hypothalamus. IL-6 levels in the CNS are negatively correlated with fat mass and this would seem to suggest a central IL-6 deficiency in obesity. *Vice versa* central administration of IL-6 increases energy expenditure and reduces fat mass in experimental animal models.

Slattery et al (58) found a significant interaction between high waist-to-hip ratio, a specific IL-6 genotype and an increased risk of breast cancer. These data suggest that IL-6 genotypes may influence breast cancer risk in conjunction with central adiposity in postmenopausal women. Moreover, a recent paper showed that the association between specific IL-6 promoter haplotype and worse outcomes in breast cancer patients was limited to those patients with ER+ tumors, thus providing further support for the hypothesis that IL-6 exerts its effect on breast cancer cells at least in part through hormonal pathways (59).

During the evolution of breast cancer, IL-6 seems to have an inhibitory action in the early-stage breast cancer, whereas high levels in advanced and metastatic breast cancer are associated with a poor prognosis due to IL-6-induced immunosuppressive activity, metabolic changes and neoplastic cell growth (60). Furthermore, IL-6 acts as a regulator of estrogen synthesis and aromatase expression and activity both in the adipose tissue and in malignant breast tissue, contributing to breast cancer progression (61). IL-6 induces cell migration through the activation of the MAPK pathway, acts as an antiapoptotic factor, promotes the osteoclasts formation and inhibits the differentiation of dendritic cells, thus facilitating the metastatic process (62).

In conclusion, IL-6 may be associated with breast cancer through several mechanisms, including regulation of insulin, inflammation and estrogen, all factors that may significantly influence the evolution of this disease (63). In fact, proinflammatory cytokines can facilitate tumor growth and metastasis by altering tumor cell biology and activating stromal cells, tumor-associated macrophages and fibroblasts (64). Systemic inflammation may also condition the vasculature in ways that enhance the extravasation, engraftment, and growth of micrometastases. Therefore, systemic chronic inflammation mediated by IL-6 may increase the risk of breast cancer recurrence and affect breast cancer prognosis (65).

OXIDATIVE STRESS

Obesity, as a result of result of metabolic and inflammatory changes, is commonly associated with increased oxidative stress, the latter characterized by high levels of reactive oxygen species (ROS) (66).

These highly reactive free radicals created by incomplete reduction of oxygen result in molecules of singlet oxygen and superoxide. Unless these free radicals are neutralized by antioxidant cell protective mechanisms, they can cause damage to lipids, proteins, and nucleic acids. ROS could also lead to progressive genetic instability, tumor progression, and metastasis in triggering the P13K/Akt pathway which in turn is activated by some of the obesity-associated cytokines and growth factors and mutagenic changes (67).

Increased oxidative stress in accumulated fat has recently been identified as an important pathologic mechanism in insulin resistance and metabolic syndrome (66). In turn, energy balance changes have marked effects on ROS levels in obse subjects: dietary energy restriction brings acute reduction in ROS, whereas overfeeding increases levels of ROS (68). Accordingly, it has been demonstrated that Common single nucleotide polymorphisms (SNPs) in candidate genes related to oxidative stress was associated with postmenopausal breast cancer risk (69).

Indeed, there is evidence that oxidative stress is involved in breast carcinogenesis. Production of ROS and nitric oxide (NO) species in cancer-associated fibroblasts is sufficient to induce genomic instability in adjacent cancer cells, via a bystander effect, potentially increasing their aggressive behavior. Breast cancer cells use "oxidative stress" in adjacent fibroblasts as an "engine" to fuel their own survival via the stromal production of nutrients. Therefore, treatment with anti-oxidants (such as N-acetyl-cysteine, metformin and quercetin) or NO inhibitors seems to be sufficient to reverse many of the cancer-associated fibroblast phenotypes (70).

INTERACTIONS BETWEEN ESTROGENS AND ADIPOKINES

Despite the involvement of estrogens in the etiology and progression of breast cancer, about 30% of these tumors do not express the ER and thus they are refractory to the antiestrogen therapy. Moreover, about 40% of breast tumors have ER but fail to respond to hormonal therapy. These findings warrant a careful assessment of the mechanism through which estrogens carry out their actions and the implication of possible alternative or synergic mechanisms capable of regulating tumorigenesis and progression of breast carcinoma.

Catalano et al (33) have demonstrated that leptin can activate the ER transcription in MCF-7 breast cancer cells independently from estradiol. Leptin induces the nuclear localization of ER through the stimulation of the synthesis of pS2, an estrogen-inducible protein, which is expressed in the estrogen-responsive breast tumor cells. These results suggest a mechanism through which leptin may have a negative action on the benefits resulting from estrogens withdrawal by the administration of aromatase inhibitors. Moreover, it has been demonstrated that leptin can directly interfere with the antiestrogenic activity and therefore with the suppression of tumor cell proliferation associated to antiestrogen drugs, in particular to fulvestrant (71). Additionally, a reciprocal functional dependency between leptin and the ER/ligand system has been found. Estrogens induced a reversible increase in leptin mRNA expression and secretion from the adipose tissue (72). It has been shown that high intratumoral levels of leptin mRNA expression in ER+ tumors are specifically involved in the growth stimulation of estrogen-dependent breast cancer through an autocrine mechanism (73). Moreover, leptin in a paracrine way induces the aromatase synthesis in the stromal cells isolated by the subcutaneous and the breast adipose tissue of premenopausal women (74). Miyoshi et al (73) hypothesized that the paracrine correlation between breast carcinoma cells and the surrounding adipose tissue is more important than the autocrine regulation. Additionally, Chen et al (75) demonstrated that tumor surgical excision did not influence circulating leptin levels in patients with breast carcinoma. This finding is consistent with the idea that the tumor leptin production is only a minor source, whereas the adipose tissue is the main contributor to its circulating levels.

Among the other adipokines, IL-6 and TNF-α also induce aromatase expression (51). In obesity the infiltration of the adipose tissue by an increased number of TNF-α and IL-6 secreting macrophages can be responsible for the increase of the estrogen synthesis from C19 steroids, thus contributing to an increased risk of breast cancer in postmenopausal obese women (76).

THERAPEUTIC PERSPECTIVES

Antiestrogens, such as tamoxifen, were the first drugs developed for the treatment of hormone-dependent breast cancer, but the third generation aromatase inhibitors have been shown to be superior to tamoxifen in terms of reducing recurrence risk and are recommended for the treatment of postmenopausal women with hormone receptor-positive breast cancer, both in the metastatic and adjuvant and neoadjuvant setting. Importantly, as the reduction in the risk of distant metastases often precedes improvements in overall survival, these results may translate into a significant survival benefit with longer follow-up. Recent studies were trying to better understand the potential influence of each adipokine on the tumorigenesis of breast cancer. In fact, a better understanding of each adipokine function may be extremely important to enable the further identification of key molecules involved in the development of breast carcinoma and to suggest new therapeutic options.

The identification of leptin and the demonstration that its circulating concentrations positively correlate with BMI have been followed by attempts to link serum leptin levels to breast cancer risk. To date, however, these studies have reported conflicting results. This is mainly because leptin was assessed indiscriminately and not in specific populations of postmenopausal rather than premenopausal patients or in patients with ER+ rather than ER-tumors. Indeed, it should be pointed out that the link between leptin and breast cancer goes through the well-known correlation of postmenopause, subsequent body weight gain, with the increase of aromatase activity and leptin levels also resulting from increased fat mass. Moreover, it is important to underline that leptin seems to have direct and specific actions on the neoplastic cell. Therefore, the role of leptin in the etiopathogenesis of breast cancer and its development would thus seem to be twofold: 1) direct and 2) indirect. In the first instance, leptin performs as a growth factor regardless of hormonal status and acts directly on its receptor present in the neoplastic cells. In the second instance, leptin levels reflect the total amount of fat mass, which can be directly correlated to the aromatasic activity and the subsequent amount of estrogens (1).

These observations are of course meaningful only for that specific subgroup of patients where increase of adipose tissue, hormone dependency, oncogenesis, tumor growth and progression are strictly correlated. In this scenario, the direct proneoplastic action of leptin is associated to aromatase hyperactivity. In this respect, great importance would be assigned to the use of aromatase inhibitors in function of the BMI and the subsequent levels of leptin. Paradoxically in obese womens we could be faced with an optimum action of the aromatase inhibitors in their capacity to suppress estrogen synthesis, but such effect could be in part counteracted by permanent high leptin levels capable of independently perform a specific stimulus of the neoplastic proliferation.

In the light of these considerations, antiestrogen and aromatase inhibitors therapy may have a different effectiveness for postmenopausal women with breast carcinoma in respect of BMI and leptin levels. A recently published exploratory analysis from the ATAC trial (77) showed that postmenopausal ER-positive breast cancer patients with a high BMI (BMI>35 kg/m2) at baseline had a significantly higher rate of breast cancer recurrence compared to those women with a low BMI (BMI < 23 kg/m2) and significantly more distant recurrences. In detail, recurrence rates in the anastrozole group were lower than those in the tamoxifen group at all BMI levels, although the benefit of anastrozole was greater in thinner women (BMI >30 kg/m2 versus BMI<28 kg/m2). One possible explanation for these findings is (as authors stated in the paper) that higher estrogen levels resulting from a high BMI may lead to incomplete inhibition with anastrozole. It seems that there are overweight/obese women whose extraglandular aromatisation from adipose tissue cannot be fully suppressed by the standard treatment dose of 1 mg/day of anastrozole. Therefore, women with a high BMI might need higher dosages to achieve the fully antitumor efficacy of this drug. To test this hypothesis a thorough assessment of BMI-related efficacy of aromatase inhibitors in randomised trials in both adjuvant and metastatic setting is warranted. Therefore, the evaluation in properly designed and adequately powered clinical trials of the potential benefit of adjusting dose of aromatase inhibitors by body weight will be critical in determining whether outcomes for overweight and obese breast cancer patients can be improved.

Moreover, as discussed in the present paper, other obesity-associated factors, including insulin, adipokines (i.e., leptin) and inflammatory mediators, may influence breast cancer growth and prognosis independently of estrogens and at least in part by interacting with estrogen signalling at a cellular level.

In particular, leptin competes with antiestrogens for the modulation of ER activity, and thus high serum levels of leptin in overweight breast cancer patients might contrast the inhibitory effects of antiestrogenic therapy on cell proliferation and ER expression and trascription. Leptin, with its capacity to increase the activation of estrogen receptors, may reduce or even overcome the antiproliferative effects induced by antiestrogen in breast carcinoma cells (71). In summary, the mass of evidence available so far seems to suggest that the increased leptin synthesis in postmenopausal overweight women may promote breast cancer growth by directly interacting with its specific receptor and by indirectly acting on the signalling pathways related to ER. Therefore, it is important to assess the use of drugs which act on the several altered pathways correlated to obesity.

Antidiabetic Drugs: Metformin

Drugs such as oral hypoglycemic agents as well as those which act on IGF-IR could be effective in reducing the insulin-mediated tumor cells growth. In the same way the adiponectine receptor agonists could be a new therapeutic approach to improve insulin-resistance and directly inhibit the proliferation of epithelial breast cells.

The concurrence of clinical and epidemiologic evidence linking hyperinsulinemia, insulin resistance, and diabetes to poor breast cancer outcomes (78) has been recently coupled with enhanced understanding of molecular effects of metformin and its potential role in malignancy (79). It is well known that insulin can promote tumorigenesis both by a direct effect on epithelial tissues, or indirectly affecting the levels of other modulators, such as insulin-like growth factors, sex hormones, and adipokines (80). The insulin/insulin-like growth factor-1 (IGF1) signaling pathway is activated when nutrients are available; *viceversa*, another alternative way is activated when cells are starved of energy through the adenosine mono-phosphate activated protein kinase (AMPK) pathway as a sensor of cellular energy balance (81). Therefore, AMPK is the central cellular energy sensor which responds to increases in the adenosine monophosphate/adenosine triphosphate ratio. Physiological conditions of nutrient deprivation activate AMPK leading to inhibition of energy-consuming processes (gluconeogenesis, protein and fatty acid synthesis, cholesterol biosynthesis) and stimulation of processes that generate energy (glycolysis, fatty acid beta oxidation), resulting in restoration of the adenosine triphosphate supply (82). One of the major growth regulatory pathways controlled by AMPK is the mammalian target of rapamycin (mTOR) pathway and its downstream substrates, such as the ribosomal S6 kinase (S6K1). This pathway regulates protein translation of cell growth regulators such as cyclin D, hypoxia inducible factor 1α (HIF1α) and MYC. All these factors control key cell processes such as: cycle progression, growth and angiogenesis (83).

Consequently, IGF signaling concurs to normal cell growth, but it is also a known mediator of the malignant phenotype. IGF1 receptor ligand binding leads to autophosphorylation of tyrosines at its kinase domain; this induces the phosphorylation of tyrosines and serines to form binding sites for insulin receptor substrates (IRS) and Src and subsequent activation of signaling via the phosphatidylinositol-3-kinase (PI3K)/Akt/mTOR and RAS/RAF/mitogen activated protein kinase (MAPK) pathways (84). It is relevant that mTOR activity is in part regulated by cellular energy levels and nutrients as well as oxygen and growth factors. When mTOR is deregulated, it leads to increased cell growth and proliferation. Therefore, on the basis of the above reports, insulin, both directly and indirectly, promotes lipid, protein, and glycogen synthesis, whereas AMPK inhibits these biosynthetic pathways.

Exciting preclinical studies have demonstrated that the antidiabetic drug metformin can inhibit the growth of cancer cells, including breast cancer, (85, 86) and population studies increasingly suggest that metformin decreases the incidence of cancer and cancer-related mortality in diabetic patients (87, 88). More recently, a retrospective study of patients who received neoadjuvant chemotherapy for breast cancer showed that diabetic cancer patients receiving metformin during their neoadjuvant chemotherapy had a higher pathological complete response rate than diabetic patients not receiving metformin (24% vs 8%, p=0.007) (89).The primary actions of metformin are inhibition of hepatic glucose production and reduction of insulin resistance in peripheral tissue leading to enhanced glucose uptake and utilisation in skeletal muscle. This reduces the levels of circulating glucose and decreases the plasma insulin levels improving long-term glycemic control and reducing the incidence of diabetes-related complications. The antineoplastic effects of metformin, and in particular in breast cancer are supported by a specific biological rationale involving important factors associated with breast cancer growth and prognosis. At cell signalling level, several mechanisms of metformin action have been proposed; the most important relates to the activation of AMPK (90).

In patients with diabetes mellitus type 2 activation of AMPK by metformin results in partial reversal of metabolic disturbances such as hyperglycaemia and insulin resistance. The beneficial effects expected from the reversal of hyperglicemia, insulin resistance and hyperinsulinemia and their mitogenic effects have indeed been demonstrated in *in vitro* and *in vivo* models of cancer. Metformin inhibits the growth of various types of cancer cells both in vitro and in vivo (85) through the activation of AMPK. Activation of AMPK by metformin results in phosphorilation and stabilisation of tuberous sclerosis complex, which integrates regulatory inputs including oxygen-dependent signals and growth factor-dependent signalling pathways such as the PI3K and the MAPK (91). Activation of AMPK by metformin can phosphorylate and activate the tumor suppressor p53 leading to the inhibition of cell division and induction of apoptosis in cells that encounter low nutrient conditions (92). This mechanism can lead to apoptosis in p53 proficient cells and induce re-expression of functional p53 in cells with low levels of wild-type p53 (93). However, p53 expression in adipose tissue is involved in the development of insulin resistance and therefore metformin-induced p53 expression may be expected to increase insulin-resistance (94).

However, the majority of the growth inhibitory effects of metformin are mediated through the inhibition of mTOR signalling (95): mTOR phosphorilates down-stream mediators leading to the regulation of cell cycle progression, cell growth and angiogenesis. Moreover, metformin reduces HER-2 protein expression in human breast cancer cells through inhibition of mTOR (96). Other reported mechanisms of action for metformin include reduced insulin-like growth factor, insulin and HER2-mediated signalling, inhibition of angiogenesis and induction of cell cycle arrest and apoptosis. Metformin may also have anti-proliferative effects both by reversing hyperinsulinaemia (97) and also by indirectly lowering IGF-I levels through effects on insulin and insulin-binding proteins levels (98).

The inhibition of angiogenesis is another proposed mechanism of metformin's effect. Metformin attenuates angiogenic stimuli in the serum of polycistic ovarian syndome patients with insulin resistance and decreases levels of vascular endothelial growth factor (VEGF) in obese diabetic patients. In addition, in vitro studies have shown inhibition of angiogenesis and inflammation by metformin through inhibition of mediators such as HIF-1α, tumor necrosis factor alpha, plasminogen activator inhibitor-1 antigen and von Willerbrand factor, possibly through the inhibition of mTOR signalling. Therefore, there is a strong preclinical rationale for a potentially beneficial effect of metformin in breast cancer outcomes.

Antiinflammatory Drugs

Since inflammation signalling pathways, through the action of some mediators such as IL-6 and TNF-α, may influence breast tumor growth and disease outcome, several studies have investigated associations between aspirin and nonsteiroidal anti-inflammatory drugs and breast cancer risk (99). A recent study demonstrated that aspirin had the greatest reduction in risk in the presence of a high-risk IL-6 genotype and a more modest effect in the presence of the lower-risk allele and concluded that the joint effect of IL-6 genotype and aspirin use attenuated the expected risk in a multiplicative way among postmenopausal women (100).

Aspirin and other NSAIDs are widely used for the treatment of minor injuries and headaches, degenerative joint diseases such as rheumatoid arthritis, and as prophylaxis against cardiovascular diseases. NSAIDs inhibit the activity of COX leading to the inhibition of synthesis of prostaglandins (PGs) that cause inflammation, swelling, pain and fever. Some NSAIDs are more potent against Cox-1 (for example, aspirin), others have greater affinity for Cox-2 (sCox-2 inhibitors).

Increasing evidence from human epidemiological studies, animal models, and in vitro experiments suggests that aspirin and other NSAIDs may prevent the occurrence of cancers of epithelial origin (101). In particular, daily intake of NSAIDs, primarily aspirin, produced risk reductions of 39% for breast cancer (102): these chemopreventive effects were apparent after 5 or more years of NSAID use and were stronger with longer duration. These observations have collectively initiated a wide variety of investigations to determine the mechanisms by which aspirin and other NSAIDs reduce the risk or progression of cancers.

In detail, research on human cell lines and animal models indicates a role for COX-2 in breast carcinogenesis (102, 103), thus suggesting that selective Cox-2 (sCox-2) inhibitors and NSAIDs may prevent the growth of mammary tumors. In fact, COX-2 is overexpressed in approximately 40% of human breast tumors and it is induced in response to stimuli such as cytokines (104).

NSAIDs may exert a protective effect against breast cancer, apart from by inhibiting Cox-2, by reducing the level of prostaglandins, estrogens and/or prolactin (105, 106). Furthermore, studies in literature suggest that in different cancer cells, aspirin induces upregulation of mitochondrial outer membrane pro-apoptotic proteins, such as Bax and Bak, and downregulation of anti-apoptotic proteins such as Bcl-2 and Bcl-xl (107) as well as increases mitochondrial membrane permeability and release of cytochrome c leading to the activation of caspases and cell apoptosis (108). One of the most widely accepted mechanisms for the anticancer effect of NSAIDs is the reduced PG synthesis through acetylation and inhibition of COX. However, NSAIDs have growth inhibitory effects against cancer cell lines that do not express COX-1 or -2 (), and against mouse embryo fibroblasts that are null for both enzymes (109, 110). These observations suggest that COX-independent pathways may also contribute to the anticancer effects of NSAIDs. Although the effects of aspirin on COX have been well-studied, little is known as to whether it induces acetylation of cellular proteins, particularly those that regulate apoptosis, which may also contribute to its anticancer effects. Alfonso et al demonstrated that the ability of aspirin to induce apoptosis involves acetylation of the tumor suppressor protein p53 (111), leading to modulation of its target genes, p21CIP1, a protein involved in cell cycle arrest, and Bax, a mitochondrial proapototic protein.

Another possible mechanism by which the COX/PGE2 cascade promotes breast cancer is via increasing estrogen production. It is known that PGE2 up-regulates aromatase activity, the enzyme that converts androgens to estrogens, leading to increased estrogen synthesis and recently, *viceversa* dose-dependent decreases of aromatase activity were observed in breast cancer cells following treatment with NSAIDs, a COX-1 selective inhibitor, and COX-2 selective inhibitors (112). Indeed, laboratory results have shown that estradiol production is decreased in breast cells exposed to the selective COX-2 inhibitor celecoxib (113). Although the above-mentioned pathway through which NSAIDs may decrease the development of breast cancer has been previously highlighted (114), the association between NSAID use and circulating estradiol in women is currently unknown. Therefore, a recent crosssectional investigation, demonstrated that NSAID use was associated with lower circulating estradiol levels in a population of postmenopausal women not taking menopausal hormone therapy (115), thus suggesting a potential mechanism through which NSAIDs exert protective effects on breast cancer.

To date, however, results of epidemiological studies of non-steroidal antiinflammatory drugs (NSAIDs) and breast cancer risk have been uncertain. In fact, several cohort studies (116-118) have found a reduced risk of breast cancer associated with aspirin use. On the other hand, others (119, 120) have failed to find any association or have even suggested an increased risk. Few meta-analyses of this association have been performed, and all have methodological limitations. None was exhaustive, and none assessed heterogeneity in an in-depth manner. However, recently an exhaustive meta-analysis on NSAID use and risk of breast cancer was carried out following the MOOSE guidelines for meta-analyses of observational studies and provided evidence that NSAID use is associated with reduced risk for breast cancer. The authors included cyclooxygenases (COX)-2 – nonselective inhibitors (a group that contains aspirin and ibuprofen as the most widely used drugs) as well as the more recent COX-2 – selective inhibitors with the aim to provide a more definitive answer about a possible inverse correlation between the use of these drugs and the risk for breast cancer (121).

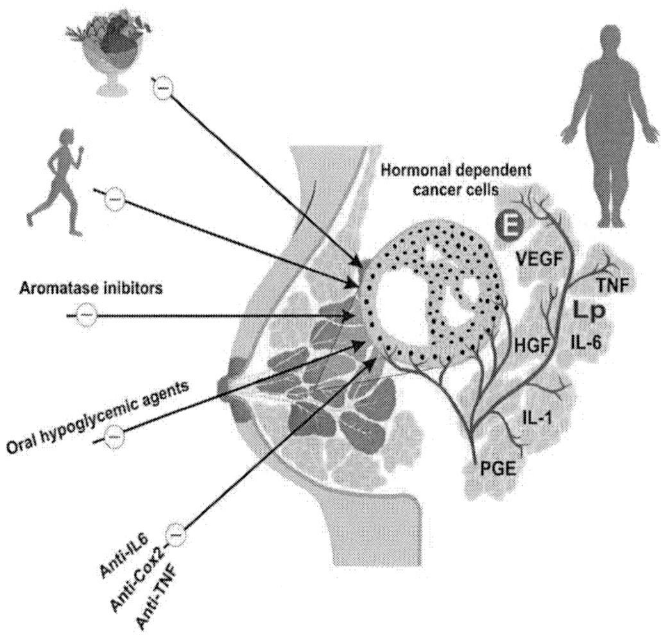

Figure 3. Potential therapeutic approaches for postmenopausal hormone-dependent breast carcinoma which develops in the context of adiposity. Adipokines, insulin, inflammation and angiogenesis-signalling pathways influence the development of hormone-dependent breast carcinoma and might represent new targets of treatment in combination with conventional hormone therapies. COX-2, cyclooxygenase-2; E, oestradiol; HGF, hepatocyte growth factor; IGF, insulin growth factor; IL, interleukin; TNF, tumor necrosis factor; VEGF, vascular endothelial growth factor.

CONCLUSION

The evidence currently available in literature would seem to suggest that the expression of adipokines as well as that of estrogens differ according to BMI changes and energy metabolic status. Therefore, a careful assessment of the nutritional status and body composition is paramount for a proper therapeutic approach for postmenopause breast carcinoma. The use of anti-diabetic and anti-inflammatory drugs associated with conventional hormone therapies and dietary/physical interventions could offer a new therapeutic approach for breast carcinoma which develops in the context of adiposity (Figure 3).

Different dietary patterns were demonstrated to influence breast cancer risk (122): in particular a food pattern characterized by high-fat food choices was significantly associated with increased risk of breast cancer. Moreover, data from epidemiological studies suggest that physical activity is important in reducing the risk of breast cancer in postmenopausal women (100). Indeed, these approaches target the upstream factors, i.e., adiposity and physical inactivity, that drive chronic inflammation linked to breast carcinogenesis and prognosis.

To date, however, only few randomized clinical trials have investigated the associations of diet, physical activity, or weight with prognosis among women diagnosed with breast cancer (123). An analysis of lifestyle and survival in the control arm of the Women's Healthy Eating and Living Study (WHEL) trial found that the combination of consuming five or more daily servings of vegetables and fruits, and accumulating $\geq$ 540 metabolic equivalent tasks-minutes/wk (equivalent to walking 30 minutes 6 days/wk), was associated with a significant survival advantage (HR, 0.56; 95% CI, 0.31 to 0.98). These findings were similar in obese and nonobese women, and were stronger in those with estrogen receptor–positive tumors. Behavior changes associated with increased physical activity have also been shown to moderately decrease cancer incidence, slow down cancer progression in model systems and improve cancer survival by multiple mechanisms, including: improved insulin resistance resulting in lower insulin levels; reduced circulating bioactive hormone concentrations resulting in increased steroid hormone binding proteins; and reduced inflammatory cytokines. Recent publications have reported on associations between physical activity after diagnosis and prognosis among breast cancer survivors. In 2,987 women from the Nurses' Health Study diagnosed with stage I to III breast cancer between 1984 and 1998 and followed until death or 2002, the relative risk of death from breast cancer for activity equivalents of walking was 0.80 for 1 to 3 hours/wk; 0.50 for 3 to 5 hours/wk; 0.56 for 5 to 8 hours/wk; and 0.60 for $\geq$ 8 hours/wk, compared with inactive women. In a cohort of 688 women diagnosed with local or regional breast cancer between 1995 and 1998 and observed until death or 2004, the HR for total deaths for women expending the energy equivalent of 2 to 3 hours/wk of brisk walking at 2 years after diagnosis was 0.33 (95% CI, 0.15 to 0.73, P for trend # .046) compared with inactive women . In a cohort of 1,970 early-stage patients with breast cancer identified primarily through a health maintenance organization, a protective association between physical activity and all-cause mortality remained in multivariable analyses (HR, 0.66;95% CI, 0.42 to 1.03; P for trend =0 .04).

Future studies that exploit emerging ways to target energy balance–responsive pathways through combinations of lifestyle (particularly diet and physical activity) and pharmacologic approaches will facilitate the translation of this research into effective cancer prevention and targeted effective therapeutic strategies in humans.

REFERENCES

[1]   Macciò, A; Madeddu, C; Mantovani, G. Adipose tissue as target organ in the treatment of hormone-dependent breast cancer: new therapeutic perspectives. *Obesity Reviews* 2009, 10, 660-670.

[2]   McTiernan, A; Irwin, M; Vongruenigen, V. Weight, physical activity, diet, and prognosis in breast and gynecologic cancers. *J Clin Oncol* 2010, 28, 4074-4080.

[3]   Dizdar, O; Alyamaç, E. Obesity: an endocrine tumor? *Med Hypotheses* 2004, 63, 790–792.

[4]   Rose, DP; Komninou, D; Stephenson, GD. Obesity, adipocytokines, and insulin resistance in breast cancer. *Obes Rev* 2004, 5, 153–165.

[5]   Bulun, SE; Lin, Z; Imir, G; Amin, S; Demura, M; Yilmaz, B; Martin, R; Utsunomiya, H; Thung, S; Gurates, B; Tamura, M; Langoi, D; Deb, S. Regulation of aromatase expression in estrogen-responsive breast and uterine disease: from bench to treatment. *Pharmacol Rev* 2005, 57, 359–383.

[6]   Harvie, M; Hooper, L; Howell, AH. Central obesity and breast cancer risk: a systematic review. *Obes Rev* 2003, 4, 157–173.

[7]   Borugian, MJ; Sheps, SB; Kim-Sing, C; Olivotto, IA; Van Patten, C; Dunn, BP; Coldman, AJ; Potter, JD; Gallagher, RP; Hislop, TG. Waist-to-hip ratio and breast cancer mortality. *Am J Epidemiology* 2003; 158:963-968.

[8]   Bulun, SE; Price, TM; Aitken, J; Mahendroo, MS; Simpson, ER. A link between breast cancer and local estrogen biosynthesis suggested by quantification of breast adipose tissue aromatase cytochrome P450 transcripts using competitive polymerase chain reaction after reverse transcription. *J Clin Endocrinol Metab* 1993, 77, 1622–1628.

[9]   Zhao, Y; Nichols, JE; Bulun, SE; Mendelson, CR; Simpson, ER. Aromatase P450 gene expression in human adipose tissue: Role of a Jak/STAT pathway in regulation of the adipose-specific promoter. *J Biol Chem* 1995, 270, 16449–16457.

[10] Zhao, Y; Agarwal, VR; Mendelson, CR; Simpson, ER. Estrogen biosynthesis proximal to a breast tumor is stimulated by PGE2 via cyclic AMP, leading to activation of promoter II of the CYP19 (aromatase) gene. *Endocrinology* 1996, 137, 5739-5742.

[11] Vona-Davis, L; Rose, DP. Adipokines as endocrine, paracrine, and autocrine factors in breast cancer risk and progression. *Endocr Relat Cancer* 2007, 14, 189–206.

[12] Vona-Davis, L; Howard-McNatt, M; Rose, DP. Adiposity, type 2 diabetes and the metabolic syndrome in breast cancer. *Obes Rev* 2007, 8, 395–408.

[13] Grundy, SM; Brewer, HB Jr; Cleeman, JI; Smith, SC Jr; Lenfant, C: National Heart, Lung, and Blood Institute, American Heart Association. Definition of metabolic syndrome: report of the National Heart, Lung, and Blood Institute/American Heart Association conference on scientific issues related to definition. *Arterioscler Thromb Vasc Biol* 2004, 24, 13–18.

[14] Godden, J; Leake, R; Kerr, DJ. The response of breast cancer cells to steroid and peptide growth factors. *Anticancer Res* 1992, 12, 1683–1688.

[15] Mawson, A; Lai, A; Carroll, JS; Sergio, CM; Mitchell, CJ; Sarcevic, B. Estrogen and insulin/IGF-1 cooperatively stimulate cell cycle progression in MCF-7 breast cancer cells through differential regulation of c-Myc and cyclin D1. *Mol Cell Endocrinol* 2005, 229, 161–173.

[16] Sachdev, D; Yee, D. The IGF system and breast cancer. *Endocr Relat Cancer* 2001, 8, 197–209.

[17] Slattery, ML; Sweeney, C; Wolff, R; Herrick, J; Baumgartner, K; Giuliano, A; Byers, T. Genetic variation in IGF1, IGFBP3, IRS1, IRS2 and risk of breast cancer in women living in Southwestern United States. *Breast Cancer Res Treat* 2007, 104, 197–209.

[18] Sachdev, D; Hartell, JS; Lee, AV; Zhang, X; Yee, D. A dominant negative type I insulin-like growth factor receptor inhibits metastasis of human cancer cells. *J Biol Chem* 2004, 279, 5017-5024.

[19] Yee, D; Lee; AV. Crosstalk between the insulin-like growth factors and estrogens in breast cancer. *J Mammary Gland Biol Neoplasia* 2000, 5, 107-115.

[20] Lorincz, AM; Sukumar, S. Molecular links between obesity and breast cancer. *Endocr Relat Cancer* 2006, 13, 279–292.

[21] McTiernan, A; Rajan, KB; Tworoger, SS; Irwin, M; Bernstein, L; Baumgartner, R; Gilliland, F; Stanczyk, FZ; Yasui, Y; Ballard-Barbash,

R. Adiposity and sex hormones in postmenopausal breast cancer survivors. *J Clin Oncol* 2003, 21, 1961–1966.

[22] Key, T; Appleby, P; Barnes, I; Reeves, G. Endogenous Hormones and Breast Cancer Collaborative Group. Endogenous sex hormones and breast cancer in postmenopausal women: reanalysis of nine prospective studies. *J Natl Cancer Inst* 2002, 94, 606–616.

[23] Catalano, MG; Frairia, R; Boccuzzi, G; Fortunati, N. Sex hormone-binding globulin antagonizes the anti-apoptotic effect of estradiol in breast cancer cells. *Mol Cell Endocrinol* 2005, 230, 31–37.

[24] Kershaw, EE; Flier, JS. Adipose tissue as an endocrine organ. *J Clin Endocrinol Metab* 2004, 89, 2548–2556.

[25] Iyengar, P; Combs, TP; Shah, SJ; Gouon-Evans, V; Pollard, JW; Albanese, C; Flanagan, L; Tenniswood, MP; Guha, C; Lisanti, MP; Pestell, RG; Scherer, PE. Adipocyte-secreted factors synergistically promote mammary tumorigenesis through induction of anti-apoptotic transcriptional programs and proto-oncogene stabilization. *Oncogene* 2003, 22, 6408-6423.

[26] Manabe, Y; Toda, S; Miyazaki, K; Sugihara, H. Mature adipocytes, but not preadipocytes, promote the growth of breast carcinoma cells in collagen gel matrix culture through cancer-stromal cell interactions. *J Pathol* 2003, 201, 221-228.

[27] Ahima, RS; Prabakaran, D; Mantzoros, C; Qu, D; Lowell, B; Maratos-Flier, E; Flier, JS. Role of leptin in the neuroendocrine response to fasting. *Nature* 1996, 382, 250–252.

[28] Simons, PJ; van den Pangaart, PS; van Roomen, CP; Aerts, JM; Boon, L. Cytokine-mediated modulation of leptin and adiponectin secretion during *in vitro* adipogenesis: evidence that tumor necrosis factor-alpha- and interleukin-1beta-treated human preadipocytes are potent leptin producers. *Cytokine* 2005, 32, 94–103.

[29] Sulkowska, M; Golaszewska, J; Wincewicz, A; Koda, M; Baltaziak, M; Sulkowski, S. Leptin-from regulation of fat metabolism to stimulation of breast cancer growth. *Pathology Oncology Research* 2006, 12, 69-72.

[30] Tessitore, L; Vizio, B; Pesola, D; Cecchini, F; Mussa, A; Argiles, JM; Benedetto, C. Adipocyte expression and circulating levels of leptin increase in both gynaecological and breast cancer patients. *Int J Oncol* 2004, 24, 1529–1535.

[31] Goodwin, PJ; Ennis, M; Fantus, IG; Pritchard, KI; Trudeau, ME; Koo, J; Hood, N. Is leptin a mediator of adverse prognostic effects of obesity in breast cancer? *J Clin Oncol* 2005, 23, 6037–6042.

[32] Yin, N; Wang, D; Zhang, H; Yi, X; Sun, X; Shi, B; Wu, H; Wu, G; Wang, X; Shang, Y. Molecular mechanisms involved in the growth stimulation of breast cancer cells by leptin. *Cancer Res* 2004, 64, 5870–5875.

[33] Catalano, S; Mauro, L; Marsico, S; Giordano, C; Rizza, P; Rago, V; Montanaro, D; Maggiolini, M; Panno, ML; Andó, S. Leptin induces, via ERK1/ERK2 signal, functional activation of estrogen receptor alpha in MCF-7 cells. *J Biol Chem* 2004, 279, 19908–19915.

[34] Hu, X; Juneja, SC; Maihle, NJ; Cleary, MP. Leptin – a growth factor in normal and malignant breast cells and for normal mammary gland development. *J Natl Cancer Inst* 2002, 94, 1704–1711.

[35] Ishikawa, M; Kitayama, J; Nagawa, H. Enhanced expression of leptin and leptin receptor (OB-R) in human breast cancer. *Clin Cancer Res* 2004, 10, 4325–4331.

[36] Fischer, S; Hanefeld, M; Haffner, SM; Fusch, C; Schwanebeck, U; Köhler, C; Fücker, K; Julius, U. Insulin-resistant patients with type 2 diabetes mellitus have higher serum leptin levels independently of body fat mass. *Acta Diabetol* 2002, 39, 105–110.

[37] Mantzoros, CS; Bolhke, K; Moschos, S; Cramer, DW. Leptin in relation to carcinoma in situ of the breast: a study of premenopausal cases and controls. *Int J Cancer* 1999, 80, 523–526.

[38] Geisler, J; Haynes, B; Ekse, D; Dowsett, M; Lønning, PE. Total body aromatization in postmenopausal breast cancer patients is strongly correlated to plasma leptin levels. *J Steroid Biochem Mol Biol* 2007, 104, 27–34.

[39] Yamauchi, T; Kamon, J; Minokoshi, Y; Ito, Y; Waki, H; Uchida, S; Yamashita, S; Noda, M; Kita, S; Ueki, K; Eto, K; Akanuma, Y; Froguel, P; Foufelle, F; Ferre, P; Carling, D; Kimura, S; Nagai, R; Kahn, BB; Kadowaki, T. Adiponectin stimulates glucose utilization and fatty-acid oxidation by activating AMP-activated protein kinase. *Nat Med* 2002, 8, 1288–1295.

[40] Matsuzawa, Y. Adiponectin: identification, physiology and clinical relevance in metabolic and vascular disease. *Atheroscler Suppl* 2005, 6, 7–14.

[41] Kadowaki, T; Yamauchi, T. Adiponectin and adiponectin receptors. *Endocr Rev* 2005, 26, 439–451.

[42] Yee, LD; Williams, N; Wen, P; Young, DC; Lester, J; Johnson, MV; Farrar, WB; Walker, MJ; Povoski, SP; Suster, S; Eng, C. Pilot study of rosiglitazone therapy in women with breast cancer: effects of short-term

therapy on tumor tissue and serum markers. *Clin Cancer Res* 2007, 13, 246–252.

[43]   Schäffler, A; Schölmerich, J; Buechler, C. Mechanisms of disease: adipokines and breast cancer-endocrine and paracrinemechanisms that connect adiposity and breast cancer. *Nature Clinical Practice* 2007, 3, 345–354.

[44]   Bråkenhielm, E; Veitonmäki, N; Cao, R; Kihara, S; Matsuzawa, Y; Zhivotovsky, B; Funahashi, T; Cao. Y. Adiponectin-induced antiangiogenesis and antitumor activity involve caspase-mediated endothelial cell apoptosis. *Proc Natl Acad Sci USA* 2004, 101, 2476–2481.

[45]   Pignatelli, M; Cocca, C; Santos, A; Perez-Castillo, A. Enhancement of BRCA1 gene expression by the peroxisome proliferatoractivated receptor gamma in the MCF-7 breast cancer cell line. *Oncogene* 2003, 22, 5446–5450.

[46]   Rehman, J; Considine, RV; Bovenkerk, JE; Li, J; Slavens, CA; Jones, RM; March, KL. Obesity is associated with increased levels of circulating hepatocyte growth factor. *J Am Coll Cardiol* 2003, 41, 1408–1413.

[47]   Sheen-Chen, SM; Liu, YW; Eng, HL; Chou, FF. Serum levels of hepatocyte growth factor in patients with breast cancer. *Cancer Epidemiol Biomarkers Prev* 2005, 14, 715–717.

[48]   Ruan, H; Lodish, HF. Insulin resistance in adipose tissue: direct and indirect effects of tumor necrosis factor-alpha. *Cytokine Growth Factor Rev* 2003, 14, 447–455.

[49]   Bulló, M; García-Lorda, P; Megias, I; Salas-Salvadó, J. Systemic inflammation, adipose tissue tumor necrosis factor, and leptin expression *Obes Res* 2003, 11, 525-531.

[50]   Coppack, SW. Pro-inflammatory cytokines and adipose tissue. *Proc Nutr Soc* 2001, 60, 349–356.

[51]   Purohit, A; Newman, SP; Reed, MJ. The role of cytokines in regulating estrogen synthesis: implications for the etiology of breast cancer. *Breast Cancer Res* 2002, 4, 65–69.

[52]   Suarez-Cuervo, C; Harris, KW; Kallman, L; Väänänen, HK; Selander, KS. Tumor necrosis factor-alpha induces interleukin-6 production via extracellular-regulated kinase 1 activation in breast cancer cells. *Breast Cancer Res Treat* 2003, 80, 71–78.

[53]   Hotamisligil, GS; Shargill, NS; Spiegelman, BM. Adipose expression of tumor necrosis factor-alpha: direct role in obesitylinked insulin

resistance. *Science* 1993, 259, 87–91.

[54]   Morley, JE; Baumgartner, RN. Cytokine-related aging process. *J Gerontol A Biol Sci Med Sci* 2004, 59, M924-M929.

[55]   Ferrari, SL; Ahn-Luong, L; Garnero, P; Humphries, SE; Greenspan, SL. Two promoter polymorphisms regulating interleukin-6 gene expression are associated with circulating levels of C-reactive protein and markers of bone resorption in postmenopausal women. *J Clin Endocrinol Metab* 2003, 88, 255–259.

[56]   Bennermo, M; Held, C; Stemme, S; Ericsson, CG; Silveira, A; Green, F; Tornvall, P. Genetic predisposition of the interleukin-6 response to inflammation: implications for a variety of major diseases? *Clin Chem* 2004, 50, 2136–2140.

[57]   Vozarova, B; Weyer, C; Hanson, K; Tataranni, PA; Bogardus, C; Pratley, RE. Circulating interleukin-6 in relation to adiposity, insulin action, and insulin secretion. *Obes Res* 2001, 9, 414–417.

[58]   Slattery, ML; Curtin, K; Sweeney, C; Wolff, RK; Baumgartner, RN; Baumgartner, KB; Giuliano, AR; Byers, T. Modifying effects of IL-6 polymorphisms on body size-associated breast cancer risk. *Obesity (Silver Spring)* 2008, 16, 339–347.

[59]   DeMichele, A; Gray, R; Horn, M; Chen, J; Aplenc, R; Vaughan, WP; Tallman, MS. Host genetic variants in the interleukin-6 promoter predict poor outcome in patients with estrogen receptor-positive, node-positive breast cancer. *Cancer Res* 2009, 69, 4184-4191.

[60]   Bachelot, T; Ray-Coquard, I; Menetrier-Caux, C; Rastkha, M; Duc, A; Blay, JY. Prognostic value of serum levels of interleukin 6 and of serum and plasma levels of vascular endothelial growth factor in hormone-refractory metastatic breast cancer patients. *Br J Cancer* 2003, 88, 1721–1726.

[61]   Purohit, A; Ghilchik, MW; Duncan, L; Wang, DY; Singh, A; Walker, MM; Reed, MJ. Aromatase activity and interleukin-6 production by normal and malignant breast tissues. *J Clin Endocrinol Metab* 1995, 80, 3052–3058.

[62]   Grano, M; Mori, G; Minielli, V; Cantatore, FP; Colucci, S; Zallone, AZ. Breast cancer cell line MDA-231 stimulates osteoclastogenesis and bone resorption in human osteoclasts. *Biochem Biophys Res Commun* 2000, 270, 1097–1100.

[63]   Slattery, ML; Curtin, K; Baumgartner, R; Sweeney, C; Byers, T; Giuliano, AR; Baumgartner, KB; Wolff, RR. IL6, aspirin, nonsteroidal anti-inflammatory drugs, and breast cancer risk in women living in the

southwestern United States. *Cancer Epidemiol Biomarkers Prev.* 2007, 16, 747–755.

[64] Cole, SW. Chronic inflammation and breast cancer recurrence. *J Clin Oncol* 2009, 27, 3418-3419.

[65] Pierce, BL; Ballard-Barbash, R; Bernstein, L; Baumgartner, RN; Neuhouser, ML, Wener, MH; Baumgartner, KB; Gilliland, FD; Sorensen, BE; McTiernan, A; Ulrich, CM. Elevated biomarkers of inflammation are associated with reduced survival among breast cancer patients. *J Clin Oncol* 2009, 27, 3437-3444.

[66] Furukawa, S; Fujita, T; Shimabukuro, M; Iwaki, M; Yamada, Y; Nakajima, Y; Nakayama, O; Makishima, M; Matsuda, M; Shimomura, I. Increased oxidative stress in obesity and its impact on metabolic syndrome. *J Clin Invest* 2004, 114, 1752-1761.

[67] Hursting, SD; Berger, NA. Energy balance, host-related factors, and cancer progression. *J Clin Oncol* 2010, 28, 4058-4065.

[68] Harvie, M; Howell, A. Energy balance adiposity and breast cancer - energy restriction strategies for breast cancer prevention. *Obesity Rev* 2006, 7, 33-47.

[69] Seibold, P; Hein, R; Schmezer, P; Hall, P; Liu, J; Dahmen, N; Flesch-Janys, D; Popanda, O; Chang-Claude, J. Polymorphisms in oxidative stress-related genes and postmenopausal breast cancer risk. *Int J Cancer* 2010, Nov 12.

[70] Martinez-Outschoorn, UE; Balliet, RM; Rivadeneira, DB; Chiavarina, B; Pavlides, S; Wang, C; Whitaker-Menezes, D; Daumer, KM; Lin, Z; Witkiewicz, AK; Flomenberg, N; Howell, A; Pestell, RG; Knudsen, ES; Sotgia, F; Lisanti, MP. Oxidative stress in cancer associated fibroblasts drives tumor-stroma co-evolution: A new paradigm for understanding tumor metabolism, the field effect and genomic instability in cancer cells. *Cell Cycle* 2010, 9, 3256-3276.

[71] Garofalo, C; Sisci, D; Surmacz, E. Leptin interferes with the effects of the antiestrogen ICI 182,780 in MCF-7 breast cancer cells. *Clin Cancer Res* 2004, 10, 6466–6475.

[72] Machinal-Quélin, F; Dieudonné, MN; Pecquery, R; Leneveu, MC; Giudicelli, Y. Direct *in vitro* effects of androgens and estrogens on ob gene expression and leptin secretion in human adipose tissue. *Endocrine* 2002, 18, 179–184.

[73] Miyoshi, Y; Funahashi, T; Tanaka, S; Taguchi, T; Tamaki, Y; Shimomura, I; Noguchi, S. High expression of leptin receptor mRNA in breast cancer tissue predicts poor prognosis for patients with high, but

not low, serum leptin levels. *Int J Cancer* 2006, 118, 1414–1419.

[74] Magoffin, DA; Weitsman, SR; Aagarwal, SK; Jakimiuk, AJ. Leptin regulation of aromatase activity in adipose stromal cells from regularly cycling women. *Ginekol Pol* 1999, 70, 1–7.

[75] Chen, DC; Chung, YF; Yeh, YT; Chaung, HC; Kuo, FC; Fu, OY; Chen, HY; Hou, MF; Yuan, SS. Serum adiponectin and leptin levels in Taiwanese breast cancer patients. *Cancer Lett* 2006, 237, 109–114.

[76] Weisberg, SP; McCann, D; Desai, M; Rosenbaum, M; Leibel, RL; Ferrante, AW Jr. Obesity is associated with macrophage accumulation in adipose tissue. *J Clin Invest* 2003, 112, 1796–1808.

[77] Sestak, I; Distler, W; Forbes, JF; Dowsett, M; Howell, A; Cuzick, J. Effect of Body Mass Index on Recurrences in Tamoxifen and Anastrozole Treated Women: An Exploratory Analysis From the ATAC Trial. *J Clin Oncol* 2010, 28, 3411-3415.

[78] Goodwin, PJ. Insulin in the adjuvant breast cancer setting: a novel therapeutic target for lifestyle and pharmacologic interventions? *J Clin Oncol* 2008, 26, 833–834.

[79] Goodwin, PJ; Ligibel, JA; Stambolic, V. Metformin in breast cancer: time for action. *J Clin Oncol* 2009, 27, 3271-3273.

[80] Calle, EE; Kaaks, R. Overweight, obesity and cancer: epidemiological evidence and proposed mechanisms. *Nat Rev Cancer* 2004, **4**, 579–591.

[81] Towel, MC; Hardie, DG. AMP-Activated Protein Kinase in Metabolic Control and Insulin Signaling. *Circulation Res* 2007, 100, 328–341.

[82] Hardie, DG. AMP-activated/SNF1 protein kinases: conserved guardians of cellular energy. *Nat Rev Cell Biol* 2007, 8, 774–785.

[83] Guertin, DA; Sabatini, DM. Defining the role of mTOR in cancer. *Cancer Cell* 2007, 12, 9–22.

[84] Gonzalez-Angulo, A; Meric-Bernstam, F. Metformin: a therapeutic opportunity in breast cancer. *Clin Cancer Res* 2010, 16, 1695-1700.

[85] Alimova, IN; Liu, B; Fan, Z; Edgerton, SM; Dillon, T; Lind, SE; Thor, AD. Metformin inhibits breast cancer cell growth, colony formation and induces cell cycle arrest in vitro. *Cell Cycle* 2009, 8, 909–915.

[86] Dowling, RJ; Zakikhani, M; Fantus, IG; Pollak, M; Sonenberg, N. Metformin inhibits mammalian target of rapamycin dependent translation initiation in breast cancer cells. *Cancer Res* 2007, 67, 10804–10812.

[87] Evans, JM; Donnelly, LA; Emslie-Smith, AM; Alessi, DR; Morris, AD. Metformin and reduced risk of cancer in diabetic patients. *BMJ* 2005, 330, 1304–1305.

[88]   Bowker, SL; Majumdar, SR; Veugelers, P; Johnson, JA. Increased cancer-related mortality for patients with type 2 diabetes who use sulfonylureas or insulin. *Diabetes Care* 2006, 29, 254–258.

[89]   Jiralerspong, S; Palla, SL; Giordano, SH; Meric-Bernstam, F; Liedtke, C; Barnett, CM; Hsu, L; Hung, MC; Hortobagyi, GN; Gonzalez-Angulo, AM. Metformin and pathologic complete responses to neoadjuvant chemotherapy in diabetic patients with breast cancer. *J Clin Oncol* 2009; **27**:3297–3302.

[90]   Zhou, G; Myers, R; Li, Y; Chen, Y; Shen, X; Fenyk-Melody, J; Wu, M; Ventre, J; Doebber, T; Fujii, N; Musi, N; Hirshman, MF; Goodyear, LJ; Moller, DE. Role of AMP-activated protein kinase in mechanism of metformin action. *J Clin Invest* 2001, 108, 1167–1174.

[91]   Inoki, K; Zhu, T; Guan, KL. TSC2 mediates cellular energy response to control cell growth and survival. *Cell* 2003, 115, 577–590.

[92]   Thoreen, CC; Sabatini, DM. AMPK and p53 help cells through lean times. *Cell Metab* 2005, 1, 287–288.

[93]   Ben Sahra, I; Laurent, K; Giuliano, S; Larbret, F; Ponzio, G; Gounon, P; Le Marchand-Brustel, Y; Giorgetti-Peraldi, S; Cormont, M; Bertolotto, C; Deckert, M; Auberger, P; Tanti, JF; Bost, F. Targeting cancer cell metabolism: the combination of metformin and 2- deoxyglucose induces p53-dependent apoptosis in prostate cancer cells. *Cancer Res* 2010, 70, 2465–2475.

[94]   Minamino, T; Orimo, M; Shimizu, I; Kunieda, T; Yokoyama, M; Ito, T; Nojima, A; Nabetani, A; Oike, Y; Matsubara, H; Ishikawa, F; Komuro, I. A crucial role for adipose tissue p53 in the regulation of insulin resistance. *Nat Med* 2009, 15, 1082–1087.

[95]   Zakikhani, M; Dowling, R; Fantus, IG; Sonenberg, N; Pollak, M. Metformin is an AMP kinase-dependent growth inhibitor for breast cancer cells. *Cancer Res* 2006, 66, 10269–10273.

[96]   Vazquez-Martin, A; Oliveras-Ferraros, C; Menendez, JA. The antidiabetic drug metformin suppresses HER2 (erbB-2) oncoprotein overexpression via inhibition of the mTOR effector p70S6K1 in human breast carcinoma cells. *Cell Cycle* 2009, 8, 88-96.

[97]   Goodwin, PJ; Pritchard, KI; Ennis, M; Clemons, M; Graham, M; Fantus, IG. Insulin-lowering effects of metformin in women with early breast cancer. *Clin Breast Cancer* 2008, 8, 501–505.

[98]   Pollak, M. Insulin and insulin-like growth factor signalling in neoplasia. *Nat Rev Cancer* 2008, 8, 915–928.

[99]   Howe, LR; Lippman, SM. Modulation of breast cancer risk by

nonsteroidal anti-inflammatory drugs. *J Natl Cancer Inst* 2008, 100, 1420-1423.

[100] Slattery, ML; Edwards, S; Murtaugh, MA; Sweeney, C; Herrick, J; Byers, T; Giuliano, AR; Baumgartner, KB. Physical activity and breast cancer risk among women in the southwestern United States. *Ann Epidemiol* 2007, 17, 342–353.

[101] Thun, MJ; Henley, SJ; Patrono, C. Non-steroidal anti-inflammatory drugs as anti-cancer agents: mechanistic, pharmacologic, and clinical issues. *J Natl Cancer Inst* 2002, 94, 252-266.

[102] Harris, RE; Beebe-Donk, J; Doss, H; Burr Doss, D. Aspirin, ibuprofen, and other non-steroidal anti-inflammatory drugs in cancer prevention: a critical review of non-selective COX-2 blockade. *Oncol Rep* 2005, 13, 559-583.

[103] Mustafa, A; Kruger, WD. Suppression of tumor formation by a cyclooxygenase-2 inhibitor and a peroxisome proliferator-activated receptor gamma agonist in an in vivo mouse model of spontaneous breast cancer. *Clin Cancer Res* 2008, 14, 4935-4942.

[104] Howe, LR. Inflammation and breast cancer. Cyclooxygenase/prostaglandin signaling and breast cancer. *Breast Cancer Res* 2007, 9, 210.

[105] Hudson, AG; Gierach, GL; Modugno, F; Simpson, J; Wilson, JW; Evans, RW; Vogel, VG; Weissfeld, JL. Nonsteroidal anti-inflammatory drug use and serum total estradiol in postmenopausal women. *Cancer Epidemiol Biomarkers Prev* 2008, 17, 680-687.

[106] Tworoger, SS; Eliassen, AH; Sluss, P; Hankinson, SE. A prospective study of plasma prolactin concentrations and risk of premenopausal and postmenopausal breast cancer. *J Clin Oncol* 2007, 25, 1482-1488.

[107] Zhou, XM; Wong, BC; Fan, XM; Zhang, HB; Lin, MC; Kung, HF; Fan, DM; Lam, SK. Non-steroidal anti-inflammatory drugs induce apoptosis in gastric cancer cells through up-regulation of bax and bak. *Carcinogenesis* 2001, 22,1393-1397.

[108] Zimmerman, KC; Waterhouse, NJ; Goldstein, JC; Schuler, M; Green, DR. Aspirin induces apoptosis through release of cytocrome c from mitochondria. *Neoplasia* 2000, 2, 505-513.

[109] Hanif, R; Pittas, A; Feng, Y; Koutsos, MI; Qiao, L; Staiano-Coico, L; Shiff, SI; Rigas, B. Effects of nonsteroidal anti-inflammatory drugs on proliferation and on apoptosis in colon cancer cells by a prostaglandin-independent pathway. *Biochem Pharmacol* 1996, 52, 237-245.

[110] Zhang, X; Morham, SG; Langenbach, R; Young, DA. Malignant

transformation and anti-neoplastic actions of nonsteroidal anti-inflammatory drugs (NSAIDs) on cyclooxygenase-null embryo fibroblasts. *J Exp Med* 1999, 190, 451-459.

[111] Alfonso, L; Srivenugopal, KS; Arumugam, TV; Abbruscato, TJ; Weidanz, JA; Bhat, GJ. Aspirin inhibits camptothecin-induced p21CIP1 levels and potentiates apoptosis in human breast cancer cells. *Int J Oncol* 2009, 34, 597-608.

[112] Brueggemeier, RW; Su, B; Sugimoto, Y; Diaz-Cruz, ES; Davis, DD. Aromatase and COX in breast cancer: enzyme inhibitors and beyond. *J Steroid Biochem Mol Biol* 2007, 106, 16–23.

[113] Prosperi, JR; Robertson, FM. Cyclooxygenase-2 directly regulates gene expression of P450 Cyp19 aromatase promoter regions pII, pI.3 and pI.7 and estradiol production in human breast tumor cells. *Prostaglandins Other Lipid Mediat* 2006, 81, 55–70.

[114] DuBois, RN. Aspirin and breast cancer prevention: the estrogen connection. *JAMA* 2004, 291, 2488 – 2489.

[115] Gierach, G; Lacey, JV Jr; Schatzkin, A; Leitzmann, MF; Richesson, D; Hollenbeck, AR; Brinton, LA. Nonsteroidal Anti-inflammatory Drug Use and Serum Total Estradiol in Postmenopausal Women (680). *Breast Cancer Research* 2008, 10; R38.

[116] Schreinemachers, DM; Everson, RB. Aspirin use and lung, colon, and breast cancer incidence in a prospective study. *Epidemiology* 1994, 5, 138–146.

[117] Harris, R; Kasbari, S; Farrar, WB. Prospective study of nonsteroidal antiinflammatory drugs and breast cancer. *Oncol Rep* 1999, 6, 71–73.

[118] Johnson, TW; Anderson, KE; Lazovich, D; Folsom, AR. Association of aspirin and nonsteroidal anti-inflammatory drug use with breast cancer. *Cancer Epidemiol Biomarkers Prev* 2002, 11,1586–1591.

[119] Marshall, SF; Bernstein, L; Anton-Culver, H. Nonsteroidal anti-inflamatory drug use and breast cancer risk by stage and hormone receptor status. *J Natl Cancer Inst* 2005, 97, 805–812.

[120] Jacobs, EJ; Thun, MJ; Bain, EB; Rodriguez, C; Henley, SJ; Calle, EE. A large cohort study of long-term daily use of adult-strength aspirin and cancer incidence. *J Natl Cancer Inst* 2007, 99, 608–615.

[121] Takkouche, B; Regueira-Méndez, C; Etminan, M. Breast Cancer and Use of Nonsteroidal Anti-inflammatory Drugs: A Meta-analysis. *J Natl Cancer Inst* 2008, 100, 1439–1447.

[122] Murtaugh, MA; Sweeney, C; Giuliano, AR; Herrick, JS; Hines, L; Byers, T; Baumgartner, KB; Slattery, ML. Diet patterns and breast

cancer risk in Hispanic and non-Hispanic white women: the Four-Corners Breast Cancer Study. *Am J Clin Nutr* 2008, 87, 978–984.

[123] McTiernan, A; Irwin, M; Vongruenigen, V. Weight, physical activity, diet, and prognosis in breast and gynecologic cancers. *J Clin Oncol* 2010, 28, 4074-4080.

In: New Trends in Body Mass Index Research   ISBN 978-1-61942-430-2
Editors: A. Vermeulen and E. De Smet   © 2012 Nova Science Publishers, Inc.

Chapter II

BODY MASS INDEX (BMI) IMPORTANCE IN PSORIASIS

S. Coimbra[1,2] and A. Santos-Silva[1,3]

[1]Instituto de Biologia Molecular e Celular (IBMC),
Universidade do Porto, Porto, Portugal
[2]Centro de Investigação das Tecnologias da Saúde (CITS),
Instituto Politécnico da Saúde Norte, CESPU, Gandra-Paredes, Portugal
[3]Departamento de Ciências Biológicas, Laboratório de Bioquímica,
Faculdade de Farmácia, Universidade do Porto, Porto, Portugal

ABSTRACT

Overweight and obesity are related with several chronic diseases, such as cardiovascular disease (CVD), and its prevalence is rapidly increasing worldwide. Body mass index (BMI) has been used as a good tool to measure obesity; however, some authors claim that it may provide surrogate information about CVD risk. Nonetheless, the value of the associations between the different anthropometric measures that could be used with CVD risk and with its risk factors are similar, providing, therefore, comparable information.

Psoriasis is a chronic inflammatory skin disease that affects about 2-3% of the population. There are several risk factors associated with psoriasis appearance, progression and severity, namely smoking, alcohol consumption, depression, repeated physical traumas and major stressful events. Moreover, psoriasis has been associated with overweight and obesity. Indeed, the prevalence of obesity in psoriatic patients seems to be higher than that observed in the general population. An average BMI of 28 to 30 kg/m^2 has been reported for psoriatic patients.

The relationship between a high BMI and psoriasis is not completely understood. Some studies refer that overweight or obesity, appear after the onset of psoriasis, while others suggest that obesity precedes and may represent a risk factor for psoriasis. The pro-inflammatory state of obesity, may, in part, explain its association with psoriasis. The release of pro-inflammatory cytokines and the altered secretion of adipokines may contribute to the pathologic changes observed in psoriasis.

The prevalence of high BMI in psoriatic patients seems to be strongly associated with an increased risk for CVD. Besides overweight/obesity, psoriasis associates with several others risk factors for CVD that might explain the prevalence of CVD events in these patients.

A high BMI may influence the therapeutic approach to psoriasis and the clinical response to treatment. Indeed, an increased BMI appears to affect negatively the initial response to treatments. In opposition, a normal or a reduction of BMI may favor/complement the treatment of psoriatic patients.

In summary, a complex relationship between BMI, psoriasis, psoriasis treatment and psoriasis morbidity and mortality exists, suggesting the need for a multidisciplinary approach in the management of patients with psoriasis. Psoriatic patients should be surveyed for both dermatological and metabolic aspects, in order to guide for the best therapy, and to monitor patients during therapy and during the inactive phase of the disease.

OVERWEIGHT AND OBESITY ACCORDING TO BMI

According to the World Health Organization (WHO), obesity affects 35% of the population (1), and its prevalence is rapidly increasing worldwide.

Obesity appears to be a consequence of an interaction between genetic and environmental factors. Considering that eating habits, with high caloric diets, sedentary lifestyle and reduced levels of physical activity contribute significantly for weight gain, and that the genetics of populations did not change significantly in the last years, the environmental component appears to be very important for the present obesity prevalence.

Body mass index (BMI) is a simple index, commonly used to classify underweight, overweight and obesity in adults, and is calculated by dividing the weight value (kg), by the square of the height (m). In adults, BMI is age

**Table 1. Body mass index (BMI) as a tool to measure body size
(Adapted from World Health Organization (1))**

	Low weight	Normal weight	Overweight	Obese I	Obese II	Obese III
BMI (kg/m^2)	< 18.5	18.5-24.9	25.0-29.9	30.0-34.9	35.0-39.9	> 40

and gender independent. Overweight and obesity is defined by a BMI between 25.0-29.9 kg/m^2, and equal or higher than 30.0 kg/m^2, respectively (Table 1). Normal weight is defined by a BMI between 18.5 and 24.9 kg/m^2. A recent report (2) estimated that for a BMI of 22.5–25.0 kg/m^2 an optimal survival is achieved, and that for moderate (BMI of 30.0-35.0 kg/m^2) and extreme obesity (BMI of 40.0-50.0 kg/m^2), a reduction in life expectancy of 3 and 10 years, respectively, occurs. Indeed, overweight and obesity are often associated with several chronic diseases, such as diabetes *mellitus* and cardiovascular diseases (CVD), becoming, therefore, a public health concern. Actually, both obesity and overweight have been associated with increased mortality (3, 4), and are known cardiovascular risk factors (5).

BMI AND OTHER ANTHROPOMETRIC INDICATORS

To evaluate body size, BMI is the anthropometric measure more used in epidemiological studies. BMI is known as a good tool to measure obesity, as BMI values correlate positively with body fat.

Obesity, is a pro-inflammatory state, usually presenting a low-grade chronic inflammation, with increased levels of several pro-inflammatory cytokines and acute phase reactants, such as tumour necrosis factor (TNF)-α, interleukin (IL)-1, IL-6 and C-reactive protein (CRP), that are positively correlated with BMI (6, 7).

There other measurements reflecting abdominal adiposity that have been highlighted, namely, waist circumference (8, 9), waist:hip ratio (10, 11) and waist:height ratio (12, 13). In the case of abdominal adiposity, the BMI value might be misleading, as individuals exhibiting a normal BMI may present a large waist circumference. The evaluation of abdominal adiposity is important due to its association with several metabolic dysfunctions, such as, glucose intolerance, reduced insulin sensitivity and adverse lipid profiles, all known as risk factors for CVD and diabetes *mellitus*.

Some authors claim that BMI provides surrogate information about CVD risk. There is no consensus about which of the anthropometric measures is the better marker for CVD risk. As referred, obesity is a strong risk factor for hypertension, dyslipidemia and diabetes *mellitus*, and all of these conditions are important cardiovascular risk factors. Some authors (14) reported that all the anthropometric indicators have similar associations with diabetes, while others (15) stated that measures of abdominal obesity were more associated with the incidence of diabetes. In another report (16), it was suggested that a small difference exists between BMI, waist circumference and waist:hip ratio, in the case of type II diabetes, but a slightly stronger association with waist:height ratio was found. For hypertension, the reports (15, 16) are consensual, as similar associations were observed between all the body size indicators and the prevalence of hypertension. For lipid profile, a study (17) in Asian and non-Asian populations, about the relationship between total cholesterol, high-density lipoprotein cholesterol, low-density lipoprotein cholesterol and triglycerides, with measures of abdominal adiposity, referred that all the measures have similar pattern, and that no single measure was superior at discriminating increased risk for dyslipidemia.

No consensus exists as to whether the measure of abdominal adiposity is a better marker for CVD risk than BMI. Indeed, in Collaboration Asia Pacific Cohort Studies (18), no clear association was found between any of the anthropometric measures with stroke outcome. In another study (19), BMI, waist circumference and waist:hip ratio were all positively associated with myocardial infarction. Although, other report (20) referred that waist:height ratio, especially in men, was more associated with CVD risk, the authors stated that the actual difference between anthropometric measures was small and unlikely to be clinically important. In accordance, Lee *et al.* (21) suggested that measures of abdominal adiposity were superior to BMI as discriminators of CVD risk, but that the differences were small and clinical irrelevant. It should be emphasized that all these studies were cross-sectional studies and, therefore, longitudinal studies are needed to clarify data. Nonetheless, considering the similar magnitude of the associations between the different anthropometric measures with CVD risk, their discriminatory ability to recognize cardiovascular risk, seems comparable.

PSORIASIS AND BMI VARIATIONS

Psoriasis is a chronic inflammatory skin disease that affects 2-3% of the population, though its prevalence varies across geographical regions of the world (22). It is characterised by an abnormal cycle of epidermal development, with epidermal hyperproliferation, altered maturation of skin cells, vascular changes and marked inflammation. The pathogenesis of the disease is still unclear, but genetic, environmental and immunologic factors appear to be involved in disease onset and in its course. There are several risk factors associated with psoriasis onset, progression and severity, namely, smoking, alcohol consumption, depression, repeated physical traumas and major stressful events.

Nowadays, it is believed that psoriasis associates with a T helper (Th)1/Th17 immune response (23). It is a complex disease in which the cytokine network is disturbed and the IL-23/Th17 axis appears to be crucial for its pathogenic mechanisms (24).

Psoriasis present some comorbidities, namely, CVD, Crohn's disease, type 2 diabetes *mellitus*, hypertension, metabolic syndrome, depression and cancer (25, 26). It has been also associated with overweight and obesity (27, 28). The prevalence of obesity in psoriatic patients seems to be higher than that observed in the general population. Henseler and Christophers (29) reported that a substantial proportion of psoriatic patients hospitalized for treatment were obese. In a case control study, involving patients with newly diagnosed psoriasis, Naldi *et al.* (28) found that the prevalence of psoriasis was two fold higher in patients with BMI > 30 kg/m^2, as compared with those with a BMI < 26 kg/m^2. This increase in obesity was also observed in the Utah psoriasis study (30). In the Lindegard study (27) and in an Italian case-control study (31) it was reported an association between psoriasis and BMI. Additionally, in the Nurses' Health Study II (32) increased obesity associated with higher risk of incidence of psoriasis.

The average BMI of psoriatic patients as been reported to be 28 to 30 kg/m^2 (33), showing that the psoriatic patient is often overweight or obese. A BMI ≥ 25.0 Kg/m^2 was included as a risk factor in the long-term prognostic risk factors for the clinical outcome of psoriasis, after diagnosis (34). Soltani-Arabshahi *et al.* (35) found that BMI in early adulthood is predictive of psoriatic arthritis, a chronic inflammatory arthropathy that occurs in association with psoriasis, probably as a consequence of the increase in inflammatory cytokines secreted by the adipose tissue and known to be associated with psoriasis.

Zhang *et al.* (36) found that buttocks, trunk, arms, leg and hand/feet were more often affected in overweight/obese psoriatic patients, probably, because those are the sites where the adipose tissue easily accumulates; these affected areas, as they are friction sites, are more prone to develop psoriasis lesions or to worsening of the lesions. The authors proposed that a gradual accumulation and expansion of adipose tissue in specific body surfaces, might account for the severity and higher risk to develop or to worsen the lesions in those sites.

Marino *et al.* (37) found a significant association between the body surface area covered with lesions and the BMI. Indeed, psoriasis severity was found to increase with obesity (38). Obesity is more prevalent in patients with severe psoriasis, as compared to patients with mild psoriasis (25). Murray *et al.* (38) found that Physician's Global Assessment (PGA) scores, an indicator of psoriasis severity, increased with BMI. An increasing effect of obesity on severity of psoriasis was also observed in Asian people (39) that was independent of age, smoke behaviour and duration of the disease and was higher in men than in women. This gender difference may be due to the fact that women and men have different distribution of body fat; men are more likely to have more visceral fat, which is known to produce several inflammatory cytokines. Takahashi *et al.* (40) observed positive significant correlations between Psoriasis Area and Severity Index (PASI) scores, another tool to evaluate psoriasis severity, and BMI, as well as between PASI and visceral adiposity.

It is not clear whether the number of patients with psoriasis and the severity of psoriasis are increasing, as the prevalence of obesity is also increasing (33).

WHAT IS THE RELATION BETWEEN PSORIASIS AND HIGH BMI?

The relationship between a high BMI, which reveals overweight or obesity, and psoriasis is not completely understood. While some studies (30, 41) establish that overweight and obesity appear after the onset of psoriasis, suggesting that obesity occurs as a consequence of the development of psoriasis, others (28, 42) found that obesity precedes and may represent a risk factor to develop psoriasis. When obesity occurs after the onset of psoriasis, it seems to contribute to the exacerbation of the disease (43).

Murray *et al.* (38) found that psoriatic patients, particularly women, were more likely to have a higher BMI. The pro-inflammatory state in psoriasis may induce a metabolic deregulation that associated with a poor quality of life and inadequate food habits, could contribute to weight gain. Indeed, it is possible that depression, eating habits, physical inactivity, alcohol consumption, stress and inflammation, often associated with psoriasis, favour the development of obesity in predisposed individuals. The Utah study (30) suggested that obesity follows psoriasis, implying that psoriasis contributes to the obese state.

Obesity may favour the onset of psoriasis, by providing a chronic level of low-grade inflammation that may contribute to trigger the development of psoriasis and may account for its severity (44). Furthermore, obesity itself, by increasing friction and trauma in the waistline and intertriginous areas, may worsen psoriasis by the Koebner phenomenon (45). Setty *et al.* (32) found a graded association between BMI and the risk of incidence of psoriasis. Conversely, a low BMI, lower than 21.0 kg/m^2, was associated with a lower risk of incidence of psoriasis. The authors (32) also observed that 30% of the psoriasis cases were attributable to a BMI $\geq$ 25.0 kg/m^2; women with a BMI $\geq$ 30.0 kg/m^2 and a BMI $\geq$ 35.0 kg/m^2, represented 50% and 63%, respectively, of the group, showing a strong association of psoriasis with excess weight. It seems that in patients weighing more than their ideal bodyweight, psoriasis is more severe, considering the involved skin area.

Nonetheless, the controversy remains: is obesity a consequence of psoriasis? Or it is the obese state that exacerbates the severity of psoriasis? Or do they coexist because they share a common underlying pathophysiology?

INFLAMMATION: A COMMON LINK

The pro-inflammatory state and impaired immunity in obesity, may, in part, explain the association of obesity with psoriasis (46). The adipose tissue is an active endocrine tissue, releasing pro-inflammatory cytokines. The increase of TNF-α, IL-1, IL-8 and IL-6 levels with obesity, may potentiate inflammation and may account for the pathologic changes observed in psoriasis. It was reported that obese individuals, as compared with non-obese, present higher blood levels of TNF-α and soluble TNF-α receptors. *In vitro* studies showed that TNF-α production is increased, and that TNF-α receptor 1 correlates with body weight, and that TNF-α receptor 2 correlates with BMI

(47). The subsets of T cell populations and their function may be reduced in human obesity, and this may be related, at least in part, to the increased TNF-α production (47).

Macrophages of the adipose tissue are likely to be an important source of pro-inflammatory cytokines. It is known that expansion of the adipose tissue during weight gain leads to a recruitment of macrophages into the adipose tissue (48). Macrophages are an important component of the non-adipocyte fraction of the adipose tissue and they are a source of adipose tissue-derived TNF-α, IL-6 and CXCL8 (49, 50). Apparently, macrophage infiltration of the white adipose tissue increases in proportion to BMI and adipocyte hypertrophy (51, 52).

Resistin is expressed by cells of the stromal compartment of the adipose tissue, particularly, by macrophages and by peripheral monocytes that are up-regulated during their differentiation to macrophages (53). High resistin levels are reported to be associated with the atherosclerotic process, and it has been shown that resistin increases the expression of several pro-inflammatory cytokines, including TNF-α and IL-6 (54). There is only a weak correlation between BMI and resistin levels (55); nonetheless, the proportion of mononuclear leucocytes within adipose tissue correlates well with BMI (48). Hyperresistinemia was already reported in psoriatic patients (53, 56).

Adipokines, such as adiponectin and leptin, may play a role in psoriasis pathogenesis, at least in the obese patients. The obese patients, especially those with visceral obesity, present decreased plasma concentrations of adiponectin that increase cardiovascular risk (43, 44). This, suggests the existence of a feedback inhibition process, working when the total body fat mass increases, that induces an increase in the secretion of other adipokines or a decrease in the metabolic function of the adipocyte (57). Adiponectin is known to inhibit the inflammatory response and to protect against metabolic diseases and CVD (55, 58). It seems to play an important role in lipid metabolism and atherogenesis. Moreover, adiponectin reduces the production of TNF-α, IL-6, interferon-γ, monocyte cell adhesion molecules, macrophage phagocytic activity and the transformation of macrophages to foam cells; it increases insulin sensitivity and the repair of damaged vasculature (43, 59). Adiponectin is considered a new emerging biomarker of cardiovascular risk (low risk for atherosclerosis and insulin resistance when adiponectin concentration is >10 µg/mL; normal risk at 7-10 µg/mL; high risk at 4-6.9 µg/mL and very high risk when <4 µg/mL) (60).

Leptin controls food intake, body weight and fat stores, and their blood levels seem to reflect the body fat mass. High levels of leptin enhance Th1 immune responses, suppress Th2 immune responses and increase macrophage activity, with production of different cytokines, namely, TNF-α and IL-6 (53, 61, 62).

In psoriatic patients low blood levels of adiponectin and high blood levels of leptin have been reported (53, 56, 61). Moreover, adiponectin presented a significant inverse correlation with BMI in psoriatic patients, and leptin presented a positive significant correlation (56). In studies in our lab (56), in a group of psoriatic patients, the prevalence of overweight/obesity was high, 71% of them presented a BMI>25 kg/m^2, and patients presented higher leptin, resistin, TNF-α and IL-6 levels, and lower adiponectin values, as compared to controls; adiponectin and leptin levels were more altered in patients with higher BMI.

HIGH BMI AS ANOTHER CVD RISK FACTOR IN PSORIASIS

Patients with psoriasis present a high frequency of CVD events and, therefore, they, usually, present CVD risk factors, such as oxidative stress, inflammation, abnormal lipid profile, overweight and obesity (41, 63-67). A pro-atherogenic lipid profile has been reported in psoriasis, that seems to worsen with the severity of psoriasis (63). Indeed, psoriasis has been considered (68) as an independent factor for dyslipidemia and for its associated complications. The higher levels of inflammatory and oxidative stress markers reported in psoriatic patients are even higher in overweight/obese psoriatic patients, and there is a correlation between them (69). Several reports (69, 70) confirm that inflammation caused by obesity and psoriasis results in increased production of reactive oxygen species through different biochemical pathways, and in impaired antioxidant status. Indeed, the prevalence of high BMI in psoriatic patients (28) seems to be strongly correlated with increased risk for CVD (5).

A high prevalence of systemic disorders obesity-related, including diabetes *mellitus*, hypertension and ischemic heart disease have been reported in psoriatic patients (29). Indeed, the risk to develop diabetes *mellitus* is slightly increased in patients with psoriasis, and this risk was higher for psoriatic patients with a longer psoriasis history, who regularly receive systemic treatment, usually used to treat the severer forms of the disease (71). Besides the high prevalence of obesity and diabetes *mellitus*, the psoriatic patients also present an increased prevalence of hypertension (25), which may also contribute to the high incidence of CVD events in psoriasis. Impaired glucose regulation, combined with hyperlipidemia (hypertriglyceridemia and reduced high-density lipoprotein cholesterol), hypertension and obesity, namely, abdominal obesity, are part of the metabolic syndrome, a pro-inflammatory state that contributes to psoriasis worsening (26, 72, 73). Some authors showed that the association of psoriasis with the metabolic syndrome is higher in the severe forms of psoriasis (25), while others refer that this association is independent of its severity (74). Obesity is a major component of the metabolic syndrome and both are important CVD risk factors. Actually, morbidity and mortality of psoriatic patients are mainly caused by cardiovascular events (41, 75). Nowadays, it is a common believe that the incidence of several CVD risk factors in psoriasis might explain the prevalence of CVD events in these patients.

The release of pro-inflammatory cytokines by the adipose tissue appears to contribute to the development of atherosclerosis and other CVDs in psoriatic obese patients. Moreover, it is known that, even in the absence of inflammatory conditions, the increased systemic inflammation in obesity induces a rise in CRP levels (76). High CRP concentrations have been reported in active psoriasis, and its values increase with psoriasis severity (77). It is known that patients with high levels of CRP exhibit an increased risk for adverse cardiovascular outcome, and, therefore, the concentration of CRP has been accepted as a good marker for risk of CVD events and mortality risk (78). Some authors believe that CRP, itself, may be an active protein in atherosclerosis (33, 79). The raised CRP in obesity may, therefore, indirectly contribute to the increased risk of CVD events in psoriatic patients.

BMI MANAGEMENT IN PSORIASIS: A FEW REMARKS

Obesity, traduced in a high BMI, may influence the therapeutic approach to the disease and the clinical response to treatment. Clinicians must be aware that the reduction of BMI, due to lifestyle modifications, may favor or complement the treatment of psoriatic patients. The treatment of obesity in psoriatic patients could be beneficial, by reducing the obesity-induced inflammation, improving the clinical outcome of the patients. Indeed, weight loss, as it may decrease the degree of inflammation induced by obesity, by lowering the levels of pro-inflammatory cytokines and macrophage infiltration in the adipose tissue (80), may be valuable for psoriasis prevention and management. Weight loss induced by life style modifications, will be accompanied by a decrease in the concentrations of TNF-α, IL-6, IL-8, CRP and of monocyte chemoattractant protein 1 (80). A very low caloric diet along 30 days induced a reduction in the levels of those cytokines (81). Moreover, the T cell dysfunction associated with obesity, can be recovered by adequate weight reduction (47). Thus, reducing obesity-induced inflammation may improve response to therapy, leading to a better clinical outcome, and, furthermore, lifestyle modifications should be recommended to the psoriatic patient with excess weight, until the ideal BMI is achieved.

Obese patients with moderate-to-severe psoriasis showed an increased response to therapy when a caloric-controlled diet was included in the treatment regimen (82), suggesting that lifestyle modifications, such as a low-caloric diet, may complement the treatment of obese psoriatic patients. Naldi et al. (31) observed an inverse correlation between fruit and fresh vegetable intake and psoriasis severity, although the total caloric intake was not evaluated in the study. Rucevic et al. (83) reported a favorable outcome in psoriatic patients after 4 weeks on a low-energy diet (855 kcal/day). It was also reported that fasting improves, at least temporarily, inflammatory conditions, including psoriasis (84, 85). In accordance with literature, diet counseling should be recommended in psoriatic patients with raised BMI, to obtain a dual benefit, for obesity/overweight and for psoriasis. Another study (45), reported a case of complete resolution of psoriasis after weight loss resulting from bariatric surgery.

After reduction to a proper body weight, patients should be encouraged to have a healthy life style, proper eating habits and exercise practice, in order to maintain the appropriate weight.

A poor response to psoriasis therapy appears to occur in heavier patients (86). According to Naldi et al. (87), the BMI affects the early clinical response to systemic treatment for psoriasis, with an increased BMI negatively affecting this response. In addition, in psoriatic patients treated with adalimumab, the PASI-50 response was observed more frequently in those with a BMI less than 30 kg/m^2, as compared to obese psoriatic patients (88).

Before a decision about the psoriatic therapy to use, it is important to consider the BMI of the patient. For instance, cyclosporine and acitretin, known to favor the development of hyperlipidemia, might not be advisable to prescribe in patients with dyslipidemia or predisposed to dyslipidemia, as the obese psoriatic patients. A fatty liver may predispose psoriatic patients to methotrexate-induced cirrhosis. Some obese patients may have their treatment courses complicated by sleep apnea, raising concern about the use of TNF inhibitors and the possible compromise of pulmonary function with the secondary development of congestive heart failure (89).

Overweight and obese patients may be more difficult to treat, due to the changes in the pharmacokinetic mechanisms of psoriatic drugs. The adipose tissue may alter the volume of distribution and, consequently, limit the efficacy of the drugs. Fixed-dose immunobiological drugs, such as, etarnecept and alefacept, appear to have their antipsoriatic effect reduced in patients with excess body weight (86, 90), probably, because the doses are inadequate for them, suggesting that perhaps a weight-adjusted dose is necessary in these cases. Interestingly, anti-TNF-α therapies used in psoriasis seem to be linked to an increase in body weight and BMI (91, 92). Esposito *et al.* (93) reported that etanercept treatment may induce weight gain and a BMI increase, and that the value of BMI do not influence the efficacy of the therapy. Cassano *et al.* (88) reported that the previous use of anti-TNF therapy did not affect *per se* the rate of responders, even though he reported a lower PASI-75 rate among the responders.

Psoriasis has been linked to a significant impairment of health related quality of life. The term quality of life, or health related quality of life, refers to a quantitative estimation of the global impact of a disease on physical, social, and psychological well-being of a patient. Psoriatic patients often manifest a variety of psychological problems, including poor self-esteem (94). Obesity represents also an insult to self-esteem and overall well-being. The coexistence of both may aggravate the quality of life of the patients and the treatment of obesity could also be beneficial from de health related quality of life perspective. On the other hand, quality of life factors, such as embarrassment and loss of self-esteem, may, by producing rises in stress levels, contribute to obesity development.

In summary, there is a complex relationship between BMI, psoriasis, psoriasis treatment and psoriasis morbidity and mortality that deserves further studies. Actually, further studies about these relations are important, not only from the public health perspective, but also for a better comprehensive management of psoriasis. Moreover, psoriatic patients may be surveyed for both dermatological and metabolic aspects. PASI is used to evaluate psoriasis severity and the affected body area; the measurement of BMI, eventually, associated with other anthropometric measures (known as markers of CVD risk), would be valuable and complement the clinical assessment of the psoriatic patient. Indeed, BMI should be used as a marker of overweight and obesity, and it should be evaluated during treatment, as it would provide useful information about efficacy and safety of treatments. Moreover its evaluation would be also valuable to guide the choice for the best therapy, for the patient. Finally, this complex interaction of psoriasis with different conditions, suggest the need for a multidisciplinary approach in the management of patients with psoriasis.

REFERENCES

[1] WOH. Obesity: Preventing and managing the global epidemic. *Report of a WHO Consultation on Obesity*. Geneve: WHO; 2000.

[2] Whitlock G, Lewington S, Sherliker P, Clarke R, Emberson J, Halsey J, et al. Body-mass index and cause-specific mortality in 900 000 adults: collaborative analyses of 57 prospective studies. *Lancet*. 2009 Mar 28;373(9669):1083-96.

[3] Cumming ME, Pinkham CA. Comparison of body mass index and waist circumference as predictors of all-cause mortality in a male insured lives population. *J Insur Med*. 2008;40(1):26-33.

[4] Shimazu T, Kuriyama S, Ohmori-Matsuda K, Kikuchi N, Nakaya N, Tsuji I. Increase in body mass index category since age 20 years and all-cause mortality: a prospective cohort study (the Ohsaki Study). *Int J Obes* (Lond). 2009 Apr;33(4):490-6.

[5] Shirai K. Obesity as the core of the metabolic syndrome and the management of coronary heart disease. *Curr Med Res Opin*. 2004 Mar;20(3):295-304.

[6] Wellen KE, Hotamisligil GS. Obesity-induced inflammatory changes in adipose tissue. *J Clin Invest*. 2003 Dec;112(12):1785-8.

[7] Panagiotakos DB, Pitsavos C, Yannakoulia M, Chrysohoou C, Stefanadis C. The implication of obesity and central fat on markers of chronic inflammation: The ATTICA study. *Atherosclerosis*. 2005 Dec;183(2):308-15.

[8] Wei M, Gaskill SP, Haffner SM, Stern MP. Waist circumference as the best predictor of noninsulin dependent diabetes mellitus (NIDDM) compared to body mass index, waist/hip ratio and other anthropometric measurements in Mexican Americans--a 7-year prospective study. *Obes Res*. 1997 Jan;5(1):16-23.

[9] Bigaard J, Frederiksen K, Tjonneland A, Thomsen BL, Overvad K, Heitmann BL, et al. Waist circumference and body composition in

relation to all-cause mortality in middle-aged men and women. *Int J Obes* (Lond). 2005 Jul;29(7):778-84.

[10] Janssen I, Katzmarzyk PT, Ross R. Waist circumference and not body mass index explains obesity-related health risk. *Am J Clin Nutr*. 2004 Mar;79(3):379-84.

[11] Welborn TA, Dhaliwal SS. Preferred clinical measures of central obesity for predicting mortality. *Eur J Clin Nutr*. 2007 Dec;61(12):1373-9.

[12] Ho SY, Lam TH, Janus ED. Waist to stature ratio is more strongly associated with cardiovascular risk factors than other simple anthropometric indices. *Ann Epidemiol*. 2003 Nov;13(10):683-91.

[13] Ashwell M, Hsieh SD. Six reasons why the waist-to-height ratio is a rapid and effective global indicator for health risks of obesity and how its use could simplify the international public health message on obesity. *Int J Food Sci Nutr*. 2005 Aug;56(5):303-7.

[14] Vazquez G, Duval S, Jacobs DR, Jr., Silventoinen K. Comparison of body mass index, waist circumference, and waist/hip ratio in predicting incident diabetes: a meta-analysis. *Epidemiol Rev*. 2007;29:115-28.

[15] Huxley R, James WP, Barzi F, Patel JV, Lear SA, Suriyawongpaisal P, et al. Ethnic comparisons of the cross-sectional relationships between measures of body size with diabetes and hypertension. *Obes Rev*. 2008 Mar;9 Suppl 1:53-61.

[16] Nyamdorj R, Qiao Q, Lam TH, Tuomilehto J, Ho SY, Pitkaniemi J, et al. BMI compared with central obesity indicators in relation to diabetes and hypertension in Asians. *Obesity* (Silver Spring). 2008 Jul;16(7):1622-35.

[17] Barzi F, Woodward M, Czernichow S, Lee CM, Kang JH, Janus E, et al. The discrimination of dyslipidaemia using anthropometric measures in ethnically diverse populations of the Asia-Pacific Region: the Obesity in Asia Collaboration. *Obes Rev*. 2010 Feb;11(2):127-36.

[18] Collaboration APCS. Central obesity and risk of cardiovascular disease in the Asia Pacific Region. *Asia Pac J Clin Nutr*. 2006;15(3):287-92.

[19] Yusuf S, Hawken S, Ounpuu S, Bautista L, Franzosi MG, Commerford P, et al. Obesity and the risk of myocardial infarction in 27,000 participants from 52 countries: a case-control study. *Lancet*. 2005 Nov 5;366(9497):1640-9.

[20] Gelber RP, Gaziano JM, Orav EJ, Manson JE, Buring JE, Kurth T. Measures of obesity and cardiovascular risk among men and women. *J Am Coll Cardiol*. 2008 Aug 19;52(8):605-15.

[21] Lee CM, Huxley RR, Wildman RP, Woodward M. Indices of abdominal obesity are better discriminators of cardiovascular risk factors than BMI: a meta-analysis. *J Clin Epidemiol.* 2008 Jul;61(7):646-53.

[22] Raychaudhuri SP, Farber EM. The prevalence of psoriasis in the world. *J Eur Acad Dermatol Venereol.* 2001 Jan;15(1):16-7.

[23] Sabat R, Philipp S, Hoflich C, Kreutzer S, Wallace E, Asadullah K, et al. Immunopathogenesis of psoriasis. *Exp Dermatol.* 2007 Oct;16(10):779-98.

[24] Coimbra S, Oliveira H, Reis F, Belo L, Rocha S, Quintanilha A, et al. Interleukin (IL)-22, IL-17, IL-23, IL-8, vascular endothelial growth factor and tumour necrosis factor-alpha levels in patients with psoriasis before, during and after psoralen-ultraviolet A and narrowband ultraviolet B therapy. *Br J Dermatol.* 2010 Dec;163(6):1282-90.

[25] Neimann AL, Shin DB, Wang X, Margolis DJ, Troxel AB, Gelfand JM. Prevalence of cardiovascular risk factors in patients with psoriasis. *J Am Acad Dermatol.* 2006 Nov;55(5):829-35.

[26] Sommer DM, Jenisch S, Suchan M, Christophers E, Weichenthal M. Increased prevalence of the metabolic syndrome in patients with moderate to severe psoriasis. *Arch Dermatol Res.* 2006 Dec;298(7):321-8.

[27] Lindegard B. Diseases associated with psoriasis in a general population of 159,200 middle-aged, urban, native Swedes. *Dermatologica.* 1986;172(6):298-304.

[28] Naldi L, Chatenoud L, Linder D, Belloni Fortina A, Peserico A, Virgili AR, et al. Cigarette smoking, body mass index, and stressful life events as risk factors for psoriasis: results from an Italian case-control study. *J Invest Dermatol.* 2005 Jul;125(1):61-7.

[29] Henseler T, Christophers E. Disease concomitance in psoriasis. J *Am Acad Dermatol.* 1995 Jun;32(6):982-6.

[30] Herron MD, Hinckley M, Hoffman MS, Papenfuss J, Hansen CB, Callis KP, et al. Impact of obesity and smoking on psoriasis presentation and management. *Arch Dermatol.* 2005 Dec;141(12):1527-34.

[31] Naldi L, Parazzini F, Peli L, Chatenoud L, Cainelli T. Dietary factors and the risk of psoriasis. Results of an Italian case-control study. *Br J Dermatol.* 1996 Jan;134(1):101-6.

[32] Setty AR, Curhan G, Choi HK. Obesity, waist circumference, weight change, and the risk of psoriasis in women: Nurses' Health Study II. *Arch Intern Med.* 2007 Aug 13-27;167(15):1670-5.

[33] Friedewald VE, Jr., Cather JC, Gordon KB, Kavanaugh A, Ridker PM, Roberts WC. The editor's roundtable: psoriasis, inflammation, and coronary artery disease. *Am J Cardiol*. 2008 Apr 15;101(8):1119-26.

[34] Sakai R, Matsui S, Fukushima M, Yasuda H, Miyauchi H, Miyachi Y. Prognostic factor analysis for plaque psoriasis. *Dermatology*. 2005;211(2):103-6.

[35] Soltani-Arabshahi R, Wong B, Feng BJ, Goldgar DE, Duffin KC, Krueger GG. Obesity in early adulthood as a risk factor for psoriatic arthritis. *Arch Dermatol*. 2010 Jul;146(7):721-6.

[36] Zhang C, Zhu KJ, Zheng HF, Cui Y, Zhou FS, Chen YL, et al. The effect of overweight and obesity on psoriasis patients in Chinese Han population: a hospital-based study. *J Eur Acad Dermatol Venereol*. Jan;25(1):87-91.

[37] Marino MG, Carboni I, De Felice C, Maurici M, Maccari F, Franco E. Risk factors for psoriasis: a retrospective study on 501 outpatients clinical records. *Ann Ig*. 2004 Nov-Dec;16(6):753-8.

[38] Murray ML, Bergstresser PR, Adams-Huet B, Cohen JB. Relationship of psoriasis severity to obesity using same-gender siblings as controls for obesity. *Clin Exp Dermatol*. 2009 Mar;34(2):140-4.

[39] Huang YH, Yang LC, Hui RY, Chang YC, Yang YW, Yang CH, et al. Relationships between obesity and the clinical severity of psoriasis in Taiwan. *J Eur Acad Dermatol Venereol*. Sep;24(9):1035-9.

[40] Takahashi H, Tsuji H, Takahashi I, Hashimoto Y, Ishida-Yamamoto A, Iizuka H. Prevalence of obesity/adiposity in Japanese psoriasis patients: adiposity is correlated with the severity of psoriasis. *J Dermatol Sci*. 2009 Jul;55(1):74-6.

[41] Mallbris L, Granath F, Hamsten A, Stahle M. Psoriasis is associated with lipid abnormalities at the onset of skin disease. *J Am Acad Dermatol*. 2006 Apr;54(4):614-21.

[42] Mallbris L, Larsson P, Bergqvist S, Vingard E, Granath F, Stahle M. Psoriasis phenotype at disease onset: clinical characterization of 400 adult cases. *J Invest Dermatol*. 2005 Mar;124(3):499-504.

[43] Sterry W, Strober BE, Menter A. Obesity in psoriasis: the metabolic, clinical and therapeutic implications. Report of an interdisciplinary conference and review. *Br J Dermatol*. 2007 Oct;157(4):649-55.

[44] Hamminga EA, van der Lely AJ, Neumann HA, Thio HB. Chronic inflammation in psoriasis and obesity: implications for therapy. *Med Hypotheses*. 2006;67(4):768-73.

[45]   Higa-Sansone G, Szomstein S, Soto F, Brasecsco O, Cohen C, Rosenthal RJ. Psoriasis remission after laparoscopic Roux-en-Y gastric bypass for morbid obesity. *Obes Surg.* 2004 Sep;14(8):1132-4.

[46]   Tanaka S, Inoue S, Isoda F, Waseda M, Ishihara M, Yamakawa T, et al. Impaired immunity in obesity: suppressed but reversible lymphocyte responsiveness. *Int J Obes Relat Metab Disord.* 1993 Nov;17(11):631-6.

[47]   Tanaka S, Isoda F, Ishihara Y, Kimura M, Yamakawa T. T lymphopaenia in relation to body mass index and TNF-alpha in human obesity: adequate weight reduction can be corrective. *Clin Endocrinol (Oxf).* 2001 Mar;54(3):347-54.

[48]   Curat CA, Wegner V, Sengenes C, Miranville A, Tonus C, Busse R, et al. Macrophages in human visceral adipose tissue: increased accumulation in obesity and a source of resistin and visfatin. *Diabetologia.* 2006 Apr;49(4):744-7.

[49]   Fain JN, Madan AK, Hiler ML, Cheema P, Bahouth SW. Comparison of the release of adipokines by adipose tissue, adipose tissue matrix, and adipocytes from visceral and subcutaneous abdominal adipose tissues of obese humans. *Endocrinology.* 2004 May;145(5):2273-82.

[50]   Bruun JM, Lihn AS, Madan AK, Pedersen SB, Schiott KM, Fain JN, et al. Higher production of IL-8 in visceral vs. subcutaneous adipose tissue. Implication of nonadipose cells in adipose tissue. *Am J Physiol Endocrinol Metab.* 2004 Jan;286(1):E8-13.

[51]   Weisberg SP, McCann D, Desai M, Rosenbaum M, Leibel RL, Ferrante AW, Jr. Obesity is associated with macrophage accumulation in adipose tissue. *J Clin Invest.* 2003 Dec;112(12):1796-808.

[52]   Curat CA, Miranville A, Sengenes C, Diehl M, Tonus C, Busse R, et al. From blood monocytes to adipose tissue-resident macrophages: induction of diapedesis by human mature adipocytes. *Diabetes.* 2004 May;53(5):1285-92.

[53]   Johnston A, Arnadottir S, Gudjonsson JE, Aphale A, Sigmarsdottir AA, Gunnarsson SI, et al. Obesity in psoriasis: leptin and resistin as mediators of cutaneous inflammation. *Br J Dermatol.* 2008 Aug;159(2):342-50.

[54]   Bokarewa M, Nagaev I, Dahlberg L, Smith U, Tarkowski A. Resistin, an adipokine with potent proinflammatory properties. *J Immunol.* 2005 May 1;174(9):5789-95.

[55]   Kaser S, Kaser A, Sandhofer A, Ebenbichler CF, Tilg H, Patsch JR. Resistin messenger-RNA expression is increased by proinflammatory

cytokines in vitro. *Biochem Biophys Res Commun.* 2003 Sep 19;309(2):286-90.

[56] Coimbra S, Oliveira H, Reis F, Belo L, Rocha S, Quintanilha A, et al. Circulating adipokine levels in Portuguese patients with psoriasis vulgaris according to body mass index, severity and therapy. *J Eur Acad Dermatol Venereol.* 2010 Dec;24(12):1386-94.

[57] Oh DK, Ciaraldi T, Henry RR. Adiponectin in health and disease. Diabetes Obes Metab. 2007 May;9(3):282-9.

[58] Takemura Y, Walsh K, Ouchi N. Adiponectin and cardiovascular inflammatory responses. *Curr Atheroscler Rep.* 2007 Sep;9(3):238-43.

[59] Fantuzzi G. Adipose tissue, adipokines, and inflammation. *J Allergy Clin Immunol.* 2005 May;115(5):911-9; quiz 20.

[60] Giannessi D, Maltinti M, Del Ry S. Adiponectin circulating levels: a new emerging biomarker of cardiovascular risk. *Pharmacol Res.* 2007 Dec;56(6):459-67.

[61] Takahashi H, Tsuji H, Takahashi I, Hashimoto Y, Ishida-Yamamoto A, Iizuka H. Plasma adiponectin and leptin levels in Japanese patients with psoriasis. *Br J Dermatol.* 2008 Nov;159(5):1207-8.

[62] Wang Y, Chen J, Zhao Y, Geng L, Song F, Chen HD. Psoriasis is associated with increased levels of serum leptin. *Br J Dermatol.* 2008 May;158(5):1134-5.

[63] Rocha-Pereira P, Santos-Silva A, Rebelo I, Figueiredo A, Quintanilha A, Teixeira F. Dislipidemia and oxidative stress in mild and in severe psoriasis as a risk for cardiovascular disease. *Clin Chim Acta. 2001* Jan;303(1-2):33-9.

[64] Coimbra S, Oliveira H, Reis F, Belo L, Rocha S, Quintanilha A, et al. Circulating levels of adiponectin, oxidized LDL and C-reactive protein in Portuguese patients with psoriasis vulgaris, according to body mass index, severity and duration of the disease. *J Dermatol Sci.* 2009 Sep;55(3):202-4.

[65] Coimbra S, Oliveira H, Reis F, Belo L, Rocha S, Quintanilha A, et al. Psoriasis therapy and cardiovascular risk factors: a 12-week follow-up study. *Am J Clin Dermatol.* 2010 Dec 1;11(6):423-32.

[66] Uyanik BS, Ari Z, Onur E, Gunduz K, Tanulku S, Durkan K. Serum lipids and apolipoproteins in patients with psoriasis. *Clin Chem Lab Med.* 2002 Jan;40(1):65-8.

[67] Vanizor Kural B, Orem A, Cimsit G, Yandi YE, Calapoglu M. Evaluation of the atherogenic tendency of lipids and lipoprotein content

and their relationships with oxidant-antioxidant system in patients with psoriasis. *Clin Chim Acta.* 2003 Feb;328(1-2):71-82.

[68] Bajaj DR, Mahesar SM, Devrajani BR, Iqbal MP. Lipid profile in patients with psoriasis presenting at Liaquat University Hospital Hyderabad. *J Pak Med Assoc.* 2009 Aug;59(8):512-5.

[69] Kaur S, Zilmer K, Kairane C, Kals M, Zilmer M. Clear differences in adiponectin level and glutathione redox status revealed in obese and normal-weight patients with psoriasis. *Br J Dermatol.* 2008 Dec;159(6):1364-7.

[70] Vincent HK, Innes KE, Vincent KR. Oxidative stress and potential interventions to reduce oxidative stress in overweight and obesity. *Diabetes Obes Metab.* 2007 Nov;9(6):813-39.

[71] Brauchli YB, Jick SS, Meier CR. Psoriasis and the risk of incident diabetes mellitus: a population-based study. *Br J Dermatol.* 2008 Dec;159(6):1331-7.

[72] Boehncke S, Thaci D, Beschmann H, Ludwig RJ, Ackermann H, Badenhoop K, et al. Psoriasis patients show signs of insulin resistance. *Br J Dermatol.* 2007 Dec;157(6):1249-51.

[73] Cohen AD, Sherf M, Vidavsky L, Vardy DA, Shapiro J, Meyerovitch J. Association between psoriasis and the metabolic syndrome. A cross-sectional study. *Dermatology.* 2008;216(2):152-5.

[74] Gisondi P, Tessari G, Conti A, Piaserico S, Schianchi S, Peserico A, et al. Prevalence of metabolic syndrome in patients with psoriasis: a hospital-based case-control study. *Br J Dermatol.* 2007 Jul;157(1):68-73.

[75] Gottlieb AB, Chao C, Dann F. Psoriasis comorbidities. *J Dermatolog Treat.* 2008;19(1):5-21.

[76] Visser M, Bouter LM, McQuillan GM, Wener MH, Harris TB. Elevated C-reactive protein levels in overweight and obese adults. *Jama.* 1999 Dec 8;282(22):2131-5.

[77] Coimbra S, Oliveira H, Reis F, Belo L, Rocha S, Quintanilha A, et al. C-reactive protein and leucocyte activation in psoriasis vulgaris according to severity and therapy. *J Eur Acad Dermatol Venereol.* 2010 Jul;24(7):789-96.

[78] Boekholdt SM, Hack CE, Sandhu MS, Luben R, Bingham SA, Wareham NJ, et al. C-reactive protein levels and coronary artery disease incidence and mortality in apparently healthy men and women: the EPIC-Norfolk prospective population study 1993-2003. *Atherosclerosis.* 2006 Aug;187(2):415-22.

[79] Yeh ET. CRP as a mediator of disease. *Circulation.* 2004 Jun 1;109(21 Suppl 1):II11-4.

[80] Bruun JM, Helge JW, Richelsen B, Stallknecht B. Diet and exercise reduce low-grade inflammation and macrophage infiltration in adipose tissue but not in skeletal muscle in severely obese subjects. *Am J Physiol Endocrinol Metab.* 2006 May;290(5):E961-7.

[81] Clement K, Viguerie N, Poitou C, Carette C, Pelloux V, Curat CA, et al. Weight loss regulates inflammation-related genes in white adipose tissue of obese subjects. *Faseb J.* 2004 Nov;18(14):1657-69.

[82] Gisondi P, Del Giglio M, Di Francesco V, Zamboni M, Girolomoni G. Weight loss improves the response of obese patients with moderate-to-severe chronic plaque psoriasis to low-dose cyclosporine therapy: a randomized, controlled, investigator-blinded clinical trial. *Am J Clin Nutr.* 2008 Nov;88(5):1242-7.

[83] Rucevic I, Perl A, Barisic-Drusko V, Adam-Perl M. The role of the low energy diet in psoriasis vulgaris treatment. *Coll Antropol.* 2003;27 Suppl 1:41-8.

[84] Lithell H, Bruce A, Gustafsson IB, Hoglund NJ, Karlstrom B, Ljunghall K, et al. A fasting and vegetarian diet treatment trial on chronic inflammatory disorders. *Acta Derm Venereol.* 1983;63(5):397-403.

[85] Kjeldsen-Kragh J, Haugen M, Borchgrevink CF, Laerum E, Eek M, Mowinkel P, et al. Controlled trial of fasting and one-year vegetarian diet in rheumatoid arthritis. *Lancet.* 1991 Oct 12;338(8772):899-902.

[86] Bardazzi F, Balestri R, Baldi E, Antonucci A, De Tommaso S, Patrizi A. Correlation between BMI and PASI in patients affected by moderate to severe psoriasis undergoing biological therapy. *Dermatol Ther.* 2010 Jan-Feb;23 Suppl 1:S14-9.

[87] Naldi L, Addis A, Chimenti S, Giannetti A, Picardo M, Tomino C, et al. Impact of body mass index and obesity on clinical response to systemic treatment for psoriasis. Evidence from the Psocare project. *Dermatology.* 2008;217(4):365-73.

[88] Cassano N, Galluccio A, De Simone C, Loconsole F, Massimino SD, Plumari A, et al. Influence of body mass index, comorbidities and prior systemic therapies on the response of psoriasis to adalimumab: an exploratory analysis from the APHRODITE data. *J Biol Regul Homeost Agents.* 2008 Oct-Dec;22(4):233-7.

[89] Buslau M, Benotmane K. Cardiovascular complications of psoriasis: does obstructive sleep apnoea play a role? *Acta Derm Venereol.* 1999 May;79(3):234.

[90] Clark L, Lebwohl M. The effect of weight on the efficacy of biologic therapy in patients with psoriasis. *J Am Acad Dermatol.* 2008 Mar;58(3):443-6.

[91] Saraceno R, Schipani C, Mazzotta A, Esposito M, Di Renzo L, De Lorenzo A, et al. Effect of anti-tumor necrosis factor-alpha therapies on body mass index in patients with psoriasis. *Pharmacol Res.* 2008 Apr;57(4):290-5.

[92] Gisondi P, Cotena C, Tessari G, Girolomoni G. Anti-tumour necrosis factor-alpha therapy increases body weight in patients with chronic plaque psoriasis: a retrospective cohort study. *J Eur Acad Dermatol Venereol.* 2008 Mar;22(3):341-4.

[93] Esposito M, Mazzotta A, Saraceno R, Schipani C, Chimenti S. Influence and variation of the body mass index in patients treated with etanercept for plaque-type psoriasis. *Int J Immunopathol Pharmacol.* 2009 Jan-Mar;22(1):219-25.

[94] Russo PA, Ilchef R, Cooper AJ. Psychiatric morbidity in psoriasis: a review. *Australas J Dermatol.* 2004 Aug;45(3):155-9; quiz 60-1.

Chapter III

INDIVIDUAL BODY TISSUE DISTRIBUTION VARIES CONSIDERABLY WITHIN AND BETWEEN ADJACENT BODY MASS INDEX CLASSIFICATIONS IN THE ELDERLY

Aldo Scafoglieri[1], Jonathan Tresignie[1], Ivan Bautmans[2], Steven Provyn[1], Erik Cattrysse[1], Peter Van Roy[1] and Jan Pieter Clarys[1]

[1] Department of Experimental Anatomy, Vrije Universiteit Brussel, Brussels, Belgium
[2] Frailty in Ageing Research Department, Vrije Universiteit Brussel, Brussels, Belgium

ABSTRACT

The body mass index (BMI) is an indicator of body composition (BC) and adiposity in particular. This status is the result of good correlations with indirect two- and three-component models predicting adiposity. The BMI has become the most widely used measure to diagnose obesity and yet no accepted ranges of fat percentage exist. Although being overweight or obese is strongly associated to excess mortality in large cohorts, the accuracy of BMI in detecting excess body adiposity in individuals is largely unknown. Moreover its direct relationship with anatomical tissues in general and subcutaneous, intra-peritoneal and intra-muscular adiposity in particular is not established. Concurrently emerging evidence indicates that health-related assessment of BC in the elderly is more appropriate if muscle mass and adiposity are considered jointly, instead of separately. However it remains unclear how BMI (weight/height^2) and/or waist circumference (WC) relate to body tissue distribution in the elderly. Therefore the relationship of BMI and WC with body tissue masses, with muscle/adipose tissue mass ratios and with trunk adipose tissue distribution was explored by direct cadaver dissection. For this purpose post-mortem whole BC and segmental adipose tissue composition of twenty-nine Belgian elderly persons (17 females and 12 males, aged 78.1±6.9 years) was determined at the anatomical tissue-system level: i.e. skin, muscle, adipose tissue, viscera and bones. Results indicate that BMI and WC are significantly related to adipose and non-adipose tissue masses in both sexes. Whole body muscle mass, and whole body and segmental adipose tissue masses correlated better with BMI (r-values between 0.61 and 0.90) than with WC (r-values between 0.49 and 0.83). BMI was also significantly and inversely related with various muscle/adipose tissue ratios in both sexes (r-values between -0.54 and -0.68), and was positively related with trunk adipose tissue distribution (i.e. ratio of internal/total body adipose tissue and ratio of internal/subcutaneous trunk adipose tissue) in elderly females (r-values between 0.50 and 0.54), but not in males. Although BMI and WC are significantly related with muscle/adipose tissue mass ratios in elderly subjects, persons with similar tissue mass proportions do not necessarily fit within the same BMI or WC risk-category. The use of BMI and/or WC for the comparison of individual BC is therefore limited, particularly in the intermediate ranges. Since individual body tissue distribution varies considerably future research should focus on adjusting BMI and WC, or on developing more valid anthropometric parameters for clinical decision making in elderly persons.

INTRODUCTION

The body mass index (BMI) and waist circumference (WC) are parameters used in the screening for and classification of overweight and obesity in adult individuals, based on their respective (apparent) correlation with total body and visceral adiposity (WHO, 2000; NIH, 1998). Although being overweight or obese is strongly associated to excess mortality in large cohorts (McGee et al., 2005; Prospective Studies Collaboration, 2009), the accuracy of the BMI in detecting excess body adiposity in individuals is largely unknown (Romero-Corral et al., 2008). Moreover generally accepted healthy percentage body fat ranges are nonexistent (Gallagher et al., 2000). Despite several meta- and mega analyses, prospective and observational BMI studies, the direct relation with anatomical tissues in general and subcutaneous, intra-peritoneal and intra-muscular adiposity in particular is not established.

Models of Body Composition Analysis

The relationships of BMI and WC with body composition (BC) is based on indirect estimations of adiposity and/or other prediction values (Baumgartner et al., 1995; Clarys et al., 1999). In fact, the validation of BMI and WC as indicators of adiposity has principally been performed against two-compartment or three-compartment models of BC such as hydrodensitometry, bioelectrical impedance analysis (BIA) or dual energy X-ray absorptiometry (DXA). These reference standards are based on predictive equations that assume constancy and/or homogeneity of the compartments without taking into account the human biological variation of tissue composition (Deurenberg, 2003; Heymsfield et al., 1997; Clarys et al., 2010, 2011). The results obtained by such models might be reasonably accurate in healthy adults, however for persons with significantly depleted muscle mass and/or bone mineral mass, the estimate of total body adiposity is inaccurate (Ellis, 2000). Ideally, validation as markers of adiposity should be performed against multi-compartment models of BC as provided by three-dimensional imaging techniques such as computed tomography (CT) and magnetic resonance imaging (MRI) or against direct measurements of adipose tissue such as total body carbon assessment and whole-body dissection (Heymsfield et al., 1997; Kvist et al., 1988; Ludesher et al., 2009). An overview of theoretical multi-compartment models which form the basis of (frequently) used methods/techniques in BC is shown in Figure1.

Even though CT and MRI are often cited as in vivo reference standards for the quantification of tissue-system level components, publications describing validation of these techniques with human cadavers are limited (Rössner et al., 1990; Janssens et al., 1994; Abate et al., 1994; Mitsiopoulos et al., 1998; Beneke et al., 1991; Engstrom et al., 1991; Hudash et al., 1985). Table 1 summarizes the available CT and/or MRI validation studies.

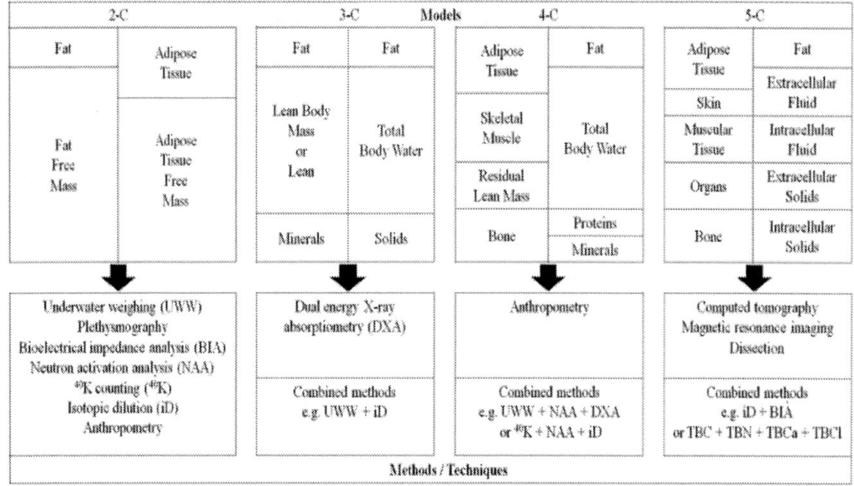

Figure 1. Theoretical multi-compartment models and BC methods/techniques used in body composition (C=compartment, TBC = total body carbon, TBN = total body nitrogen, TBCa = total body calcium, TBCl = total body chlorine).

Table 1. Overview of CT and MRI validation studies with human cadaver material

Author	subjects	CT	MRI	tissue quantity	ROI
Hudash et al. 1985	1	X		AT / muscle / bone - CSA	thigh
Rössner et al. 1990	2	X		AT - CSA	abdomen
Beneke et al. 1991	1		X	muscle - CSA	thigh
Engstrom et al. 1991	3	X	X	muscle - CSA	thigh
Abate et al. 1994	3		X	AT mass	abdomen
Janssens et al. 1994	6	X		AT / muscle / bone - CSA AT / muscle / bone - VOL	arm - leg - trunk
Mitsiopoulos et al. 1998	2	X	X	AT / muscle - CSA AT / muscle - VOL	arm - leg

CT = computed tomography, MRI = magnetic resonance imaging, ROI = region of interest, AT = adipose tissue, CSA = cross sectional area, VOL = volume.

Body Composition Changes in the Elderly

Emerging evidence indicates that health-related assessment of BC in the elderly is more appropriate if muscle mass and adiposity are considered jointly, instead of separately (Zamboni et al., 2008; Rolland et al., 2009). In this context, BMI has been suggested as a powerful indicator of muscle mass in elderly persons (as determined by DXA) (Iannuzzi-Sucich et al., 2002). Sarcopenia, defined as age-related loss of skeletal muscle mass, creates a major BC change that contributes to a large percentage of disability with increasing age (Bautmans et al., 2009; Janssen et al., 2002). In parallel, ageing is accompanied by an increase in visceral adiposity, which is a known risk factor for morbidity and mortality, even when the total amount of adipose tissue (AT) remains constant (Zamboni et al., 1997) (Figure 2).

Because adipose tissue replaces lean tissue with increasing age, older subjects tend to present a greater proportion of adipose tissue compared to younger individuals with the same BMI (Baumgartner et al., 1995; Elia, 2001). Regardless the mechanisms underlying these changes, it remains unclear how BMI and WC relate to direct BC measures in the elderly. Therefore this chapter aimed to explore the relationship of BMI and WC with body tissue masses, with muscle/adipose tissue mass ratios and with trunk adipose tissue distribution, based on an anatomical 5-compartment model obtained by dissection of cadavers of elderly persons.

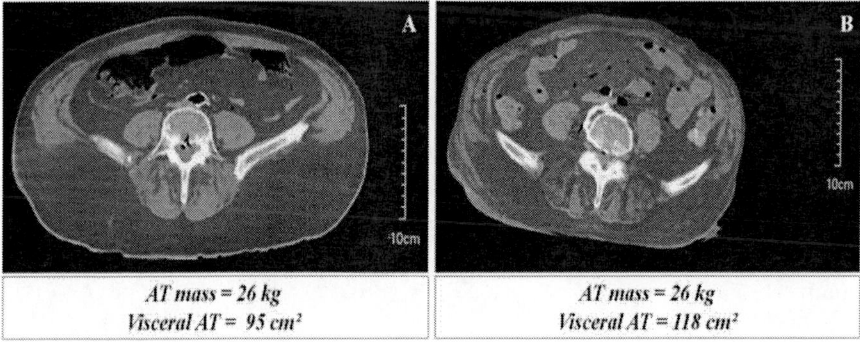

Figure 2. Computed tomography slices of the abdomen at L5 level in two old males matched for total body adipose tissue (AT) mass (26 kg). The visceral AT area (i.e. AT within the abdominal cavity) is higher in male B (118 cm²) compared to male A (95 cm²).

PROCEDURES

By means of a will system, adult Belgian citizens can donate their bodies for medical and scientific research purposes to the university of their choice. All data were collected in the Department of Anatomy at the Vrije Universiteit Brussel (Brussels, Belgium) during separate whole-body dissection projects known as the Brussels Cadaver Analysis Study (BCAS) (Clarys et al., 1984, 1999; Janssens et al., 1994). Data from twenty-nine well-preserved white Caucasian cadavers of subjects aged 65 years and over (17 female and 12 male) are reported here. The most common cause of death of the subjects was heart disease (Table 2).

Out of one BCAS project 14 female and 9 male cadavers were included, with a mean age of 77.5 ± 6.9 years (Clarys et al., 1984, 1999). Data from three male and three female additional cadavers with a mean age of 80.7 ± 6.8 years were obtained from another BCAS dissection project (Janssens et al., 1994; Clarys et al., 1999). All cadavers were embalmed within 48 hours after death. All applicable institutional, governmental and legal regulations concerning the ethical approval of human volunteers were followed during the dissection projects.

Anthropometry

The CAS project provided anthropometric measures allowing for the calculation of BMI and waist circumference (WC). Supine length was measured with the cadaver on a horizontal surface, using a custom-made anthropometer. BMI was calculated as weight divided by height squared

Table 2. Causes of death[*] of the subjects

	Females	Males
Natural	5	6
Heart attack	6	4
Stroke	1	0
Accident	1	0
Cancer	2	1
Renal insufficiency	1	0
Respiratory insufficiency	0	1
Leukemia	1	0

[*] official diagnose on death certificate.

(kg/m^2). For ease of measurement, the cadaver was suspended by an adapted orthopaedic head harness, and manipulated by a pulley attached to the ceiling. Waist circumference (the smallest girth between the iliac crest and the costal border) was measured with a flexible metal tape ruler to the nearest 0.1 cm. All measurements were performed with the cadaver warmed to ambient temperature (24°C) in order to limit temperature-related differences in texture and mobility of the skin and subcutaneous AT.

Calculation of Tissue Masses and Definitions

The cadavers were weighed immediately before dissection, which started in the early morning and continued until completion (± 14-20h later). All cadavers were dissected into their various components expressed on the tissue-level system i.e. skin, muscle, adipose tissue, viscera and bones; which were weighed to the nearest 0.001kg with dehydration reduced to a minimum (Wang et al., 1992). Detailed methodology of dissection procedures has been reported elsewhere (Clarys et al., 1984, 1999; Martin et al., 2003). The evaporative loss of body fluid during the dissection was calculated as the difference between total body weight before dissection and total tissue weight after dissection. The individual loss in each cadaver was allocated back to the different tissues in proportion to their respective masses. After this correction, the sum of the weights of all dissected tissues was equal to the cadaver's whole body weight prior to dissection.

Six body segments were defined: the four limbs, trunk and head. For the trunk segmental AT weights were recorded as follows: total trunk adipose tissue mass being the sum of trunk subcutaneous adipose tissue mass (SAT) and trunk internal adipose tissue mass (IAT, the sum of intra-abdominal AT (i.e. visceral and retroperitoneal AT) and intra-thoracic AT). For the limbs segmental AT masses were calculated: upper limbs adipose tissue mass and lower limbs adipose tissue mass. Finally total subcutaneous adipose tissue mass was computed (i.e. the difference between AT and IAT).

We considered three measures of muscle to adipose tissue proportions: the ratio of muscle mass to AT, the ratio of muscle mass to IAT and the ratio of muscle mass to SAT. We also calculated two measures of regional trunk adipose tissue proportion: the ratio of IAT to AT and the ratio of IAT to SAT.

Table 3. Physical characteristics and body composition of the subjects

	Female (n = 17) Mean ± SD (range)	Male (n = 12) Mean ± SD (range)
Physical characteristics		
Age (years)	79.9 ± 7.1 (68-94)	75.6 ± 6.1 (65-87)
Weight (kg)	58.8 ± 11.6 (32.0-75.4)	61.7 ± 14.9 (38.5-85.7)
Height (cm)	1.59 ± 0.07 (1.46-1.73)	1.67 ± 0.06 (1.60-1.80)[†]
BMI (kg/m^2)	23.4 ± 4.6 (12.9-30.9)	21.9 ± 4.3 (14.7-28.4)
Underweight (n)	2	2
Normal weight (n)	9	7
Overweight (n)	4	4
Obese (n)	1	0
WC (cm)	80.4 ± 7.3 (69.7-94.0)	83.4 ± 7.0 (73.1-94.3)
Low-risk (n)	9	10
Moderate-risk (n)	6	1
High-risk (n)	2	1
Whole body composition		
Total body AT (kg)	23.2 ± 8.9 (4.6-40.1)	16.4 ± 6.8 (5.7-25.7)[*]
Skin (kg)	3.2 ± 0.6 (1.7-4.1)	3.5 ± 0.7 (2.5-4.7)
Muscle (kg)	17.1 ± 3.2 (12.2-23.4)	22.5 ± 6.2 (14.0-34.8)[†]
Bone (kg)	7.7 ± 0.8 (6.7-10.0)	9.6 ± 1.5 (7.4-12.6)[‡]
Viscera (kg)	7.5 ± 1.4 (5.8-10.7)	9.8 ± 3.2 (6.3-18.9)[*]
Segmental body composition		
Total trunk AT (kg)	10.7 ± 4.6 (2.7-19.2)	8.4 ± 3.9 (3.2-14.2)
trunk subcutaneous AT (kg)	7.6 ± 3.1 (2.5-13.4)	5.4 ± 2.7 (2.6-10.4)
trunk internal AT (kg)	3.1 ± 1.7 (0.3-5.8)	3.0 ± 1.6 (0.5-5.3)
Upper limbs AT (kg)	2.2 ± 0.8 (0.4-3.7)	1.3 ± 0.6 (0.3-2.4)[†]
Lower limbs AT (kg)	9.7 ± 4.1 (1.2-17.5)	6.2 ± 2.5 (1.7-9.5)[*]
Head AT (kg)	0.5 ± 0.2 (0.3-0.9)	0.5 ± 0.2 (0.3-0.8)
Total body subcutaneous AT (kg)	19.7 ± 7.6 (3.3-34.3)	12.8 ± 5.6 (3.7-20.9)[*]
Body composition ratio's		
Muscle/AT	0.90 ± 0.53 (0.36-2.70)	1.56 ± 0.57 (0.65-2.46)[†]
Muscle/IAT	9.4 ± 10.8 (2.4-46.2)	10.7 ± 7.7 (3.1-26.9)
Muscle/SAT	2.7 ± 1.2 (1.0-5.0)	4.9 ± 1.8 (2.0-9.1)[†]
IAT/AT (%)	12.6 ± 3.5 (5.3-17.6)	17.6 ± 5.3 (9.1-24.8)[†]
IAT/SAT (%)	40.5 ± 15.5 (10.9-73.9)	58.9 ± 27.9 (18.8-116.9)[*]

n = number of subjects, BMI = body mass index, WC = waist circumference, AT = total body adipose tissue, IAT = Trunk internal adipose tissue, SAT = Trunk subcutaneous adipose tissue. [*]$p<0.05$, [†]$p<0.01$, [‡]$p<0.001$.

Statistical Data Analysis and Graphical Representation

Statistical Package for Social Sciences (version 17.0.1 for Windows, SPSS Inc, Chicago, USA) was used for the data analysis. Data are reported as mean ± standard deviation. Normality of data distributions was verified using Kolmogorov-Smirnov Goodness of Fit test (p>0.05). Gender differences in BC were calculated using unpaired t-tests. The relationships of BMI and WC with BC constituents were assessed using Pearson correlation coefficients. For illustrative purposes, subjects were classified according to BMI based on the International Classification of adult underweight (BMI ≤ 18.5 kg/m²), overweight (BMI ≥ 25 kg/m2) and obesity (BMI ≥ 30 kg/m2) as defined by the WHO (2000). Females and males were also classified in low-risk (females, < 80 cm; males, < 94 cm), moderate-risk (females, ranging from 80 cm to 88 cm; males, ranging from 94 cm to 102 cm) and high-risk (females, ≥ 88 cm; males, ≥ 102 cm) WC categories as proposed by Lean and colleagues (1995).

Table 4. Pearson correlation coefficients for the relationships of BMI and WC with absolute tissue masses in 17 female and 12 male cadavers by dissection

	BMI		WC	
	Female	Male	Female	Male
Whole body tissue masses				
Adipose tissue	0.80[‡]	0.84[†]	0.67[†]	0.70[*]
Skin	0.76[‡]	0.83[†]	0.76[‡]	0.61[*]
Muscle	0.68[†]	0.89[‡]	0.50[*]	0.71[†]
Bone	-0.05	0.42	0.14	0.57
Viscera	0.47	0.54	0.57[*]	0.79[†]
Segmental AT masses				
Total trunk AT	0.69[†]	0.82[†]	0.61[*]	0.76[†]
trunk subcutaneous AT	0.61[†]	0.78[†]	0.62[†]	0.83[†]
trunk internal AT	0.72[†]	0.68[*]	0.49[*]	0.44
Upper limbs AT	0.90[‡]	0.81[†]	0.81[‡]	0.46
Lower limbs AT	0.77[‡]	0.78[†]	0.61[*]	0.57
Head AT	0.40	0.24	0.31	0.35
Total body subcutaneous AT	0.81[‡]	0.85[‡]	0.69[†]	0.66[*]

BMI = body mass index, WC = waist circumference, AT = adipose tissue, [*]p<0.05, [†]p<0.01, [‡]p<0.001.

DIRECT RELATIONSHIPS OF BMI AND WC WITH BODY COMPOSITION

Total body weight (BW) for the whole sample before dissection was 60.0 ± 12.9 kg. Evaporative loss of fluid (ELF) during dissection was 2.0 ± 0.6 kg and the accuracy of the whole-body dissection method (ELF/BW) ranged from 0.6% to 6.8% (mean = 3.3 ± 1.3%).

Compared to female, male were significantly taller (p<0.01) and showed lower total body and segmental AT masses (p<0.05), higher muscle (p<0.01), bone (p<0.001) and visceral tissue masses (p<0.05); higher muscle to AT ratio's and muscle to SAT ratio (p<0.01), and higher proportions of IAT (p<0.01) (see Table 3). No significant gender differences were found for age, weight, BMI and WC.

Relation to Whole Body and Segmental Tissue Masses

BMI and WC were significantly and positively related to various tissue masses in both sexes (Table 4). Muscle tissue, skin tissue, whole body and segmental AT correlated better with BMI (r-values between 0.61 and 0.90) than with WC (r-values between 0.49 and 0.83). SAT correlated equally well with BMI (r-values between 0.61 and 0.78) and with WC (r-values between 0.62 and 0.83). Visceral mass correlated better with WC (r-values between 0.57 and 0.79) than with BMI (p>0.05).

Relation to Muscle Tissue Mass Proportions

Both in females and in males BMI was significantly and inversely related with ratios of muscle mass to AT masses. Both muscle tissue mass and AT masses increase with BMI in a quasi-linear manner; their ratio, however, decreases with increasing BMI. Visual inspection of the graphs in Figures 3 to 5 reveals major differences in muscle tissue mass proportions according to gender and WHO cutoff-values for BMI.

For example, the ratio of muscle mass to AT mass ranged from 0.5 to 2.5 in males with normal BMI-values (Figure 3). On the other hand similar values for muscle to adipose tissue ratio's were found in females classified within different BMI-categories, ranging from underweight to obese.

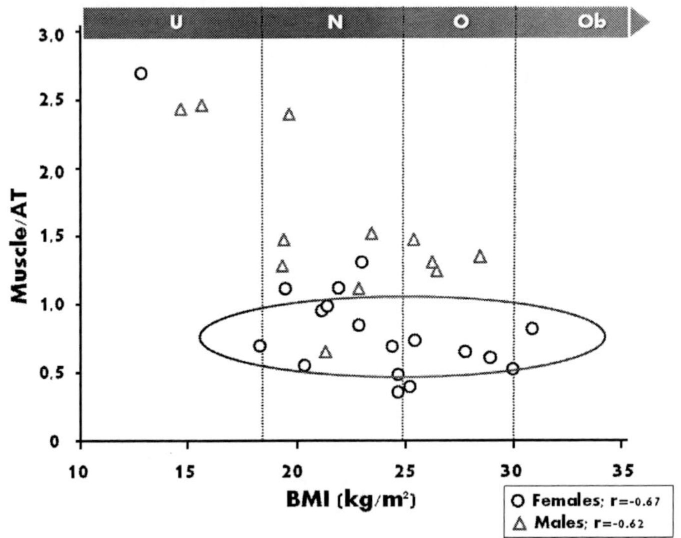

Figure 3. Direct relationship of BMI with the ratio of muscle to adipose tissue (AT) in 29 elderly cadavers (U=underweight, BMI<18.5; N=normal weight, 18.5≤BMI<25; O=overweight, 25≤BMI<30; Ob=obese, BMI≥30).

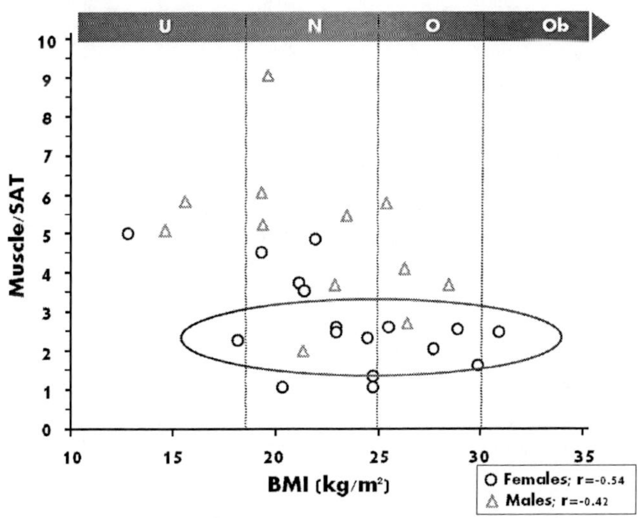

Figure 4. Direct relationship of BMI with the ratio of muscle to trunk subcutaneous adipose tissue (SAT) in 29 elderly cadavers (U=underweight, BMI<18.5; N=normal weight, 18.5≤BMI<25; O=overweight, 25≤BMI<30; Ob=obese, BMI≥30).

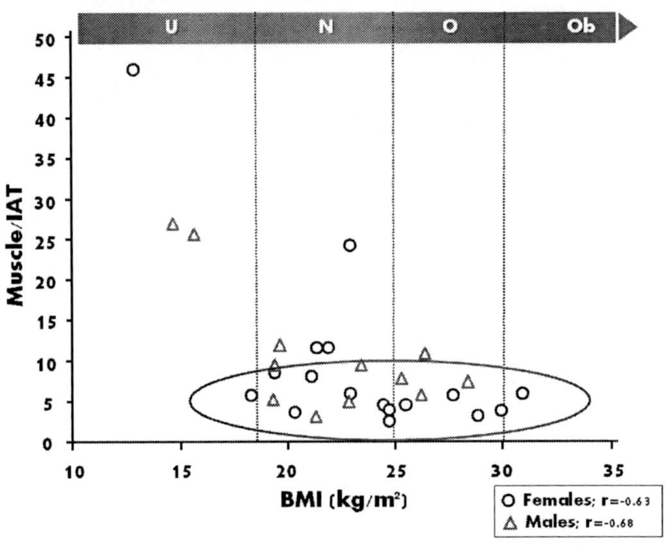

Figure 5. Direct relationship of BMI with the ratio of muscle to trunk internal adipose tissue (IAT) in 29 elderly cadavers (U=underweight, BMI<18.5; N=normal weight, 18.5≤BMI<25; O=overweight, 25≤BMI<30; Ob=obese, BMI≥30).

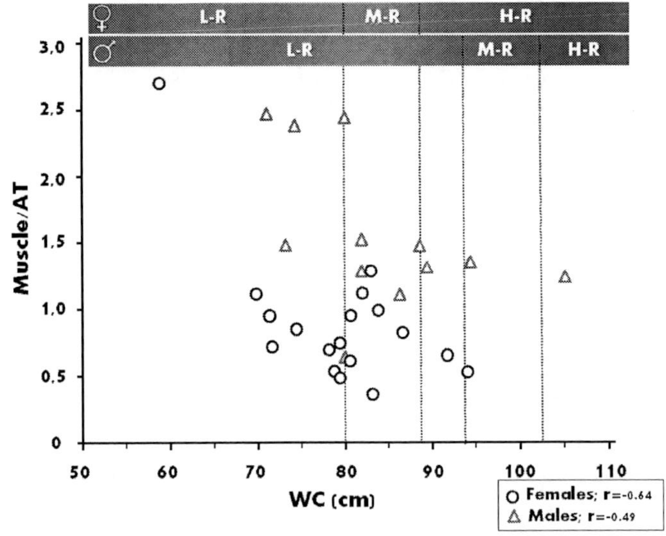

Figure 6. Direct relationship of WC with the ratio of muscle to adipose tissue (AT) in 29 elderly cadavers (female categories: L-R = low-risk, WC<80cm; M-R = moderate-risk, 80cm≤WC<88cm; H-R = high-risk, WC≥88cm; male categories: L-R = low-risk, WC<94cm; M-R = moderate-risk, 94cm≤WC<102cm; H-R = high-risk, WC≥102cm).

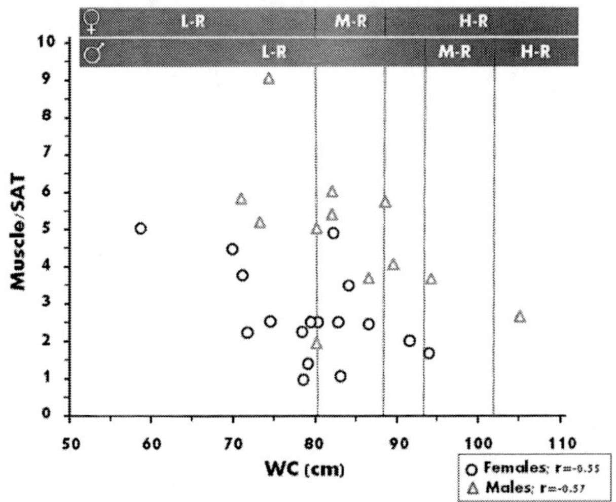

Figure 7. Direct relationship of WC with the ratio of muscle to trunk subcutaneous adipose tissue (SAT) in 29 elderly cadavers (female categories: L-R = low-risk, WC<80cm; M-R = moderate-risk, 80cm≤WC<88cm; H-R = high-risk, WC≥88cm; male categories: L-R = low-risk, WC<94cm; M-R = moderate-risk, 94cm≤WC<102cm; H-R = high-risk, WC≥102cm).

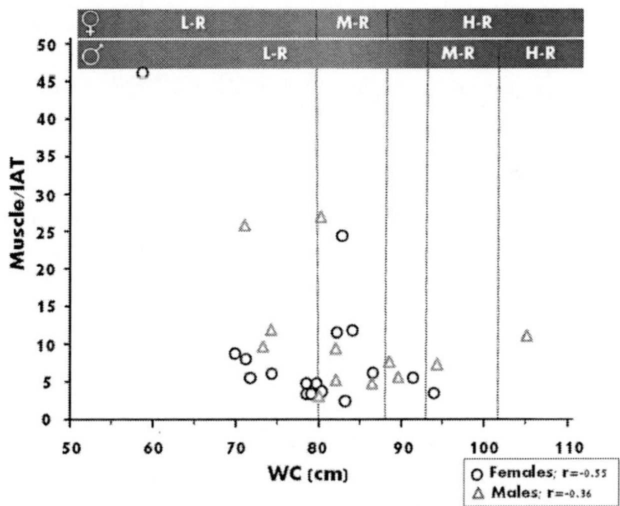

Figure 8. Direct relationship of WC with the ratio of muscle to trunk internal adipose tissue (IAT) in 29 elderly cadavers (female categories: L-R = low-risk, WC<80cm; M-R = moderate-risk, 80cm≤WC<88cm; H-R = high-risk, WC≥88cm; male categories: L-R = low-risk, WC<94cm; M-R = moderate-risk, 94cm≤WC<102cm; H-R = high-risk, WC≥102cm).

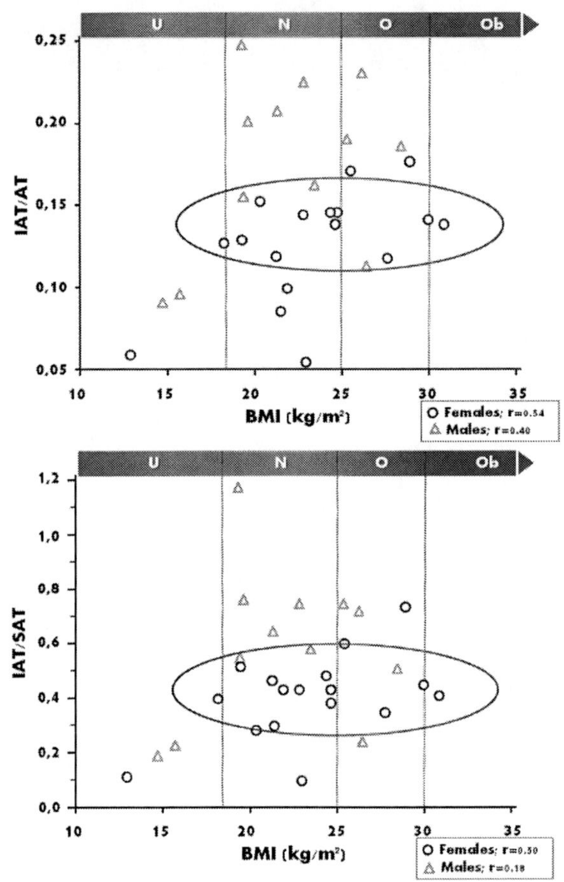

Figure 9. Direct relationship of BMI with trunk adipose tissue distribution in 29 elderly cadavers (U=underweight, BMI<18.5; N=normal weight, 18.5≤BMI<25; O=overweight, 25≤BMI<30; Ob=obese, BMI≥30, AT = adipose tissue, IAT = trunk internal AT, SAT = trunk subcutaneous AT).

The ratio of muscle mass to IAT mass was not significantly different in subjects with normal BMI compared to those presenting an elevated BMI.

Waist circumference correlated significantly and inversely with ratios of muscle mass to AT masses in females, but not in males (Figures 6-8). Visual inspection of the graphs in Figures 6 to 8 reveals important differences in muscle tissue mass proportions based on WC categories, similar to those found based on BMI-classification. This is not surprising given the fact that BMI and WC are highly correlated both in females (r=0.77; p<0.001) and in males (r=0.91; p<0.001).

Relation to Trunk Adipose Tissue Distribution

BMI correlated significantly to measures of trunk adipose tissue proportions in females, but not in males ($p<0.05$; Figure 9). Waist circumference was not significantly related to the ratio of IAT to AT nor to the ratio of IAT to SAT in our sample ($p>0.05$). Visual inspection of the graphs in Figure 9 shows that trunk AT distribution varies considerably between sexes and within BMI-categories. For example, the ratio of IAT to SAT was not different between normal weight and overweight females.

CLINICAL RELEVANCE

Understanding the relationship between BMI, WC and BC in the elderly may provide better interpretation of these measures in clinical practice (Bedogni et al., 2001). The exact determination of the muscle and adipose tissue compartments is difficult in living humans, and mainly based on 'reference' BC methods such as CT or MRI (Abate et al., 1994; Mitsiopoulos et al., 1998). To our knowledge, this is the first report relating BMI and WC to directly obtained measurements of the muscle and adipose tissue compartments in elderly subjects (Martin et al., 2003).

The design of the procedure described in this chapter is unique in the sense that it requires no assumptions regarding the measurement and the calculation of the BC constituents. It has been showed that moderate to strong relationships of BMI and WC with absolute tissue masses and with muscle tissue mass proportions in elderly subjects exist. These results confirm the findings of previous validation work using CT and MRI on living subjects (Kvist et al., 1988; Ludesher et al., 2009; Lee et al., 2000; Ferrannini et al., 2008). However cautious clinical interpretation is warranted since important inter-individual differences in tissue proportions were found in subjects with similar BMI and/or WC values.

Body Mass Index and Waist Circumference Categories: Measures of Body Tissue Distribution in the Elderly?

Sarcopenic-obesity has been defined as a condition in elderly persons reflected by low muscle mass (sarcopenia) in combination with high AT mass (obesity) (Zamboni et al., 2008). Although it is unclear which clinical condition, sarcopenia or obesity, may precede in the development of sarcopenic-obesity, it is suggested that the age-related increase in adipose tissue mass generally precedes the loss of skeletal muscle mass (Rolland et al., 2009). Body mass index and WC may offer the clinician a practical anthropometric measurement for assessing a subject's whole body and visceral AT content. Sex specific differences in BC were found, elderly females proportionally having more adipose tissue than males of similar age and BMI, who in turn are more muscular. Consequently the ratio of muscle mass to total body adipose tissue mass was found to be significantly higher in males compared to females. The observation that BMI is significantly and inversely related to the ratio of muscle to total body AT mass for both sexes, might validate the association of BMI with the lean/fat ratio as determined by BIA (Ozenoglu et al., 2009). It has to be pointed out that the significant inverse relationship between BMI and the measures of muscle mass distribution in this sample may result from the high muscle tissue proportions of the individuals classified as underweight. It has been suggested previously that regional muscle/AT ratio is closely related to aging and to visceral AT accumulation (Kitajima et al., 2009). Interestingly and in contrast to the sex specific differences in total body adiposity and muscularity, internal adipose tissue mass was not different between females and males in our sample. Since the latter represents a major metabolic compartment within the body, this observation might be of great importance. Although BMI is related to IAT, it has to be pointed out that important inter-individual differences within and between adjacent WHO-classifications do exist. Elderly individuals with similar BMI-values do not necessarily present similar levels of internal adiposity. This observation might jeopardize the clinical interpretation of the association between BMI and BC compartments based on BMI alone. These results suggest that additional assessment (such as imaging methods) may be indicated in order to quantify this important metabolic compartment. In this context, it has been suggested that ultrasound is able to account for visceral adiposity (Martin et al., 2003).

Can Simple Anthropometric Measures Detect Inter-Individual Differences in Trunk Composition?

Besides the determination of absolute AT quantities, its distribution within the body is an important health consideration (Baumgartner et al., 1995). It is well known that visceral AT concentration carries greater cardiovascular health risk compared to subcutaneous AT accumulation (Larsson et al., 1992). Visceral AT and subcutaneous AT can predict different health-risks, based on their own morphological and functional features, even for a given level of abdominal adiposity (Sniderman et al., 2007). Visceral AT has been repeatedly linked to an increased risk of dyslipidemia, dysglycemia and vascular disease. By contrast, subcutaneous AT has been associated with better metabolic outcomes. In this chapter sex specific differences in trunk adipose tissue distribution were described. Elderly males showed lower AT mass but higher proportions of internal AT compared to females of similar age and BMI. This observation validates previous findings as determined by MRI (Ferrannini et al., 2008). In our sample BMI was positively related to regional AT distribution in females only, suggesting that BMI-values do not allow distinction between internal and subcutaneous adipose tissue accumulation in elderly males. This is partly in agreement with the findings of Seidell et al. (1987) who found no significant correlations between BMI and the ratio of visceral to subcutaneous adipose tissue area using CT in a younger population. Waist circumference is generally accepted as a practical measurement for assessing a subject's visceral adipose tissue content. However, since WC is a composite measure of visceral and subcutaneous adipose tissue, it might not distinguish visceral from subcutaneous adipose tissue. Moreover WC was also significantly related to visceral mass suggesting a lack of discriminatory power of WC to differentiate between adipose and non-adipose tissue. To our knowledge, no recent studies are available reporting the relationship of WC with trunk AT distribution (as defined in the present manuscript). In the present chapter, WC was not significantly correlated to measures of trunk AT distribution, such as the ratio of IAT to SAT. It should also be observed that WC was a better correlate of SAT than of IAT in both sexes, suggesting that WC might be a more appropriate indicator of subcutaneous than of internal adiposity, in particular in elderly males. This observation supports previous findings using MRI in vivo (Ferrannini et al., 2008). These results indicate that inter-individual differences in trunk adipose tissue composition might not be detected by simple anthropometric measures such as BMI or WC, in particular in elderly persons.

Limitations of Dissection Procedure

The 'reference' method for the determination of BC was cadaver dissection. Although this method has limitations including tissue dehydration, an age matched in vivo and post mortem constitutional and anthropometric comparison has shown an overall similarity of macroscopic characteristics between subjects (Clarys et al., 2006). Since no data are available on the duration of the clinical-pathologic status of the subjects, it remains unclear to which extent body composition might have been affected in the chronically ill subjects (n=6). On the other hand, it has to be pointed out that adiposity indices such as BMI and WC are regularly used in the evaluation and follow-up of the nutritional status both in healthy elderly and in patients. The precision of our method to determine BC averaged 3.3%, which indicates that dehydration and/or losses of material during the dissection procedures were negligible. It is therefore unlikely that the method of choice biased the results presented here. Moreover the mean difference between actual weight and CT derived or MRI estimated weight reaches 5.6% to 6.0%, the latter being considered as a gold standard method in BC (Baumgartner et al., 1995; Heymsfield et al., 1997). An inevitable restriction proper to a whole-body dissection is the relatively limited number of individuals whose BC can be determined. This is due to the work-related insensitivity of the dissection procedures and the limited availability of subjects. Therefore results reported here should preferably be confirmed in a larger sample.

CONCLUSION

It is suggested that BMI and WC are significantly related with whole body and segmental adipose tissue masses and with several ratios of muscle to adipose tissue in elderly subjects. However persons with similar tissue mass proportions do not necessarily fit within the same BMI or WC risk-category. The use of BMI and/or WC for the comparison of individual BC is therefore limited, particularly in the intermediate ranges. Since BMI and WC are composite measures of BC, assessment of important metabolic body compartments themselves is warranted in elderly persons. Future research should focus on adjusting BMI and WC, or on developing more valid anthropometric parameters for clinical decision making in elderly persons.

REFERENCES

Abate, N; Burns, D; Peshock, RM; Garg, A; Grundy, SM. Estimation of adipose tissue mass by magnetic resonance imaging: validation against dissection in human cadavers. *Journal of Lipid Research*, 1994, 35, 1490-1496.

Baumgartner, RN; Heymsfield, SB; Roche, AF. Human body composition and the epidemiology of chronic disease. *Obesity Research*, 1995, 3, 73-95.

Bautmans, I; Van Puyvelde, K; Mets, T. Sarcopenia and functional decline: pathophysiology, prevention and therapy. *Acta Clinica Belgica*, 2009, 64, 303-316.

Bedogni, G; Pietrobelli, A; Heymsfield, SB; Borghi, A; Manzieri, AM; Morini, P; Battistini, N; Salvioli, G. Is body mass index a measure of adiposity in elderly women? *Obesity Research*, 2001, 9, 17-20.

Beneke, R; Neuerburg, J; Bohndorf, K. Muscle cross-section measurement by magnetic resonance imaging. European Journal of Applied Physiology and Occupational Physiology, 1991, 63, 424-9.

Clarys, JP; Martin, AD; Drinkwater, DT. Gross tissue weights in the human body by cadaver dissection. *Human Biology*, 1984, 56, 459-473.

Clarys, JP; Martin, AD; Marfell-Jones, M; Janssens, V; Caboor, D; Drinkwater, DT. Human body composition: A review of adult dissection data. *American Journal of Human Biology*, 1999, 11, 167-174.

Clarys, JP; Provyn, S; Marfell-Jones, M; Van Roy, P. Morphological and constitutional comparison of age-matched in-vivo and post-mortem populations. *Morphologie,* 2006, 90, 189-196.

Clarys, JP; Scafoglieri, A; Provyn, S; Louis, O; Wallace, JA; De Mey, J. A macro-quality evaluation of DXA variables using whole dissection, ashing and computer tomography in pigs. *Obesity*, 2010, 18, 1477-1485.

Clarys, JP; Scafoglieri, A; Provyn, S; Sesboüé, B; Van Roy, P. Hazards of hydrodensitometry. *Journal of Sports Medicine and Physical Fitness*, 2011, 51, 95-102.

Deurenberg, P. Validation of body composition methods and assumptions. *British Journal of Nutrition*, 2003, 90, 485-486.

Elia, M. Obesity in the elderly. *Obesity Research*, 2001, 9, 244S-248S.

Ellis, KJ. Human body composition: in vivo methods. Physiological Reviews, 2000, 80, 649-80.

Engstrom, CM; Loeb, GE; Reid, JG; Forrest, WJ; Avruch, L. Morphometry of the human thigh muscles. A comparison between anatomical sections and computer tomographic and magnetic resonance images. *Journal of Anatomy*, 1991, 176, 139-56.

Ferrannini, E; Sironi, AM; Iozzo, P; Gastaldelli, A. Intra-abdominal adiposity, abdominal obesity, and cardiometabolic risk. *European Heart Journal Supplements*, 2008, 10, B4–B10.

Gallagher, D; Heymsfield, SB; Heo, M; Jebb, SA; Murgatroyd, PR; Sakamoto, Y.

Healthy percentage body fat ranges: an approach for developing guidelines based on body mass index. Am J Clin Nutr, 2000, 72, 694-701

Heymsfield, SB; Wang, Z; Baumgartner, RN; Ross, R. Human body composition: advances in models and methods. *Annual Review of Nutrition*, 1997, 17, 527-558.

Hudash, G; Albright, JP; McAuley, E; Martin, RK; Fulton, M. Cross-sectional thigh components: computerized tomographic assessment. *Medicine in Science Sports & Exercise,* 1985, 17, 417-21.

Iannuzzi-Sucich, M; Prestwood, KM; Kenny, AM. Prevalence of sarcopenia and predictors of skeletal muscle mass in healthy, older men and women. *The Journals of Gerontology. Series A, Biological Sciiences and Medical Sciences*, 2002, 57, M772-777.

Janssen, I; Heymsfield, SB; Ross, R. Low relative skeletal muscle mass (sarcopenia) in older persons is associated with functional impairment and physical disability. *Journal of the American Geriatrics Society*, 2002, 50, 889-896.

Janssens, V; Thys, P; Clarys, JP; Kvist, H; Chowdhury, B; Zinzen, E; Cabri, J. Post-mortem limitations of body composition analysis by computed tomography. *Ergonomics*, 1994, 37, 207-216.

Kitajima, Y; Eguchi, Y; Ishibashi, E; Nakashita, S; Aoki, S; Toda, S; Mizuta, T; Ozaki, I; Ono, N; Eguchi, T; Arai, K; Iwakiri, R; Fujimoto, K. Age-related fat deposition in multifidus muscle could be a marker for nonalcoholic fatty liver disease. *Journal of Gastroenterology,* 2010, 45, 218-24.

Kvist, H; Chowdhury, B; Grangard, U; Tylén, U; Sjöström, L. Total and visceral adipose tissue volumes derived from measurements with computed tomography in adult men and women: predictive equations. *American Journal of Clinical Nutrition*, 1988, 48, 1351-1361.

Larsson, B; Bengtsson, C; Björntorp, P; Lapidus, L; Sjöström, L; Svärdsudd, K; Tibblin, G; Wedel, H; Welin, L; Wilhelmsen, L. Is abdominal body fat distribution a major explanation for the sex difference in the incidence of myocardial infarction? The study of men born in 1913 and the study of women, Göteborg, Sweden. *American Journal of Epidemiology,* 1992, 135, 266-273.

Lean, MEJ; Han, TS; Morrison, CE. Waist circumference as a measure for indicating need for weight management. *BMJ*, 1995, 311, 158-161.

Lee, RC; Wang, Z; Heo, M; Ross, R; Janssen, I; Heymsfield, SB. Total-body skeletal muscle mass: development and crossvalidation of anthropometric prediction models. *American Journal of Clinical Nutrition*, 2000, 72, 796-803.

Ludesher, B; Machann, J; Eschweiler, GW; Vanhöfen, S; Maenz, C; Thamer, C; Claussen, CD; Schick, F. Correlation of fat distribution in whole body MRI with generally used anthropometric data. *Investigative Radiology*, 2009, 44, 712-719.

Martin, AD; Daniel, M; Clarys, JP; Marfell-Jones, MJ. Cadaver-assessed validity of anthropometric indicators of adipose tissue distribution. *International Journal of Obesity Related Metabolic Disorders*, 2003, 27, 1052-1058.

Martin, AD; Janssens, V; Caboor, D; Clarys, JP; Marfell-Jones, MJ. Relationships between visceral, trunk and whole-body adipose tissue weights by cadaver dissection. *Annals of Human Biology,* 2003, 30, 668-677.

McGee, DL; Diverse Populations Collaboration. Body mass index and mortality: a meta-analysis based on person-level data from twenty-six observational studies. *Annals of Epidemiology,* 2005, 15, 87-97.

Mitsiopoulos, N; Baumgartner, RN; Heymsfield, SB; Lyons, W; Gallagher, D; Ross, R. Cadaver validation of skeletal muscle measurement by magnetic resonance imaging and computerized tomography. *Journal of Applied Physiology,* 1998, 85, 115-122.

National Institutes of Health, National Heart, Lung, and Blood Institute. Clinical guidelines on the identification, evaluation, and treatment of overweight and obesity in adults: the evidence report. *Obesity Research*, 1998, 6, S51-S210.

Obesity: preventing and managing the global epidemic. Report of a WHO consultation. *World Health Organisation Technical Report Series,* 2000, 894, 1-253.

Ozenoglu, A; Ugurlu, S; Can, G; Hatemi, H. Reference values of body composition for adult females who are classified as normal weight, overweight or obese according to body mass index. *Endocrine Regulations*, 2009, 43, 29-37.

Prospective Studies Collaboration; Whitlock, G; Lewington, S; Sherliker, P; Clarke, R; Emberson, J; Halsey, J; Qizilbash, N; Collins, R; Peto, R. Body-mass index and cause-specific mortality in 900 000 adults: collaborative analyses of 57 prospective studies. *Lancet,* 2009, 373, 1083-96.

Rolland, Y; Lauwers-Cances, V; Cristini, C; Abellan van Kan, G; Janssen, I; Morley, JE; Vellas, B. Difficulties with physical function associated with obesity, sarcopenia, and sarcopenic-obesity in community-dwelling elderly women: the EPIDOS (EPIDemiologie de l'OSteoporose) Study. *American Journal of Clinical Nutrition,* 2009, 89, 1895-1900.

Romero-Corral, A; Montori, VM; Somers, VK; Korinek, J; Thomas, RJ; Allison, TG; Mookadam, F; Lopez-Jimenez, F. Association of bodyweight with total mortality and with cardiovascular events in coronary artery disease: a systematic review of cohort studies. *Lancet,* 2006, 368, 666-78.

Rössner, S; Bo, WG; Hiltbrandt, E; Hinson, W; Karstaedt, N; Santago, P; Sobol, WT; Crouse, JR. Adipose tissue determinations in cadavers: A comparison between cross-sectional planimetry and computed tomography. *International Journal of Obesity,* 1990, 14, 839-902.

Seidell, JC; Oosterlee, A; Thijssen, MA; Burema, J; Deurenberg, P; Hautvast, JG; Ruijs, JH. Assessment of intra-abdominal and subcutaneous abdominal fat: relation between anthropometry and computed tomography. *American Journal of Clinical Nutrition,* 1987, 45, 7-13.

Sniderman, AD; Bhopal, R; Prabhakaran, D; Sarrafzadegan, N; Tchernof, A. Why might South Asians be so susceptible to central obesity and its atherogenic consequences? The adipose tissue overflow hypothesis. *International Journal of Epidemiology,* 2007, 36, 220-225.

Wang, ZM; Pierson, RN Jr; Heymsfield, SB. The five-level model: a new approach to organizing body-composition research. *American Journal of Clinical Nutrition,* 1992, 56, 19-28.

Zamboni, M; Armellini, F; Harris, T; Turcato, E; Micciolo, R; Bergamo-Andreis, IA; Bosello, O. Effects of age on body fat distribution and cardiovascular risk factors in women. *American Journal of Clinical Nutrition,* 1997, 66, 111-115.

Zamboni, M; Mazzali, G; Fantin, F; Rossi, A; Di Francesco, V. Sarcopenic obesity: a new category of obesity in the elderly. *Nutrition, Metabolism, and Cardiovascular Diseases: NMCD,* 2008, 18, 388-395.

Chapter IV

AGE AND SEX VARIATIONS IN BODY MASS INDEX AND CHRONIC ENERGY DEFICIENCY AMONG ADULT SANTALS OF PURULIA DISTRICT, WEST BENGAL, INDIA

Subal Das and Kaushik Bose

Department of Anthropology, Vidyasagar University, Midnapore,
West Bengal, India

ABSTRACT

This chapter was a cross-sectional one, undertaken to determine the prevalence of undernutrition using body mass index among 18 years and above Santali adults of Purulia District, West Bengal, India. A total of 791 (345 males and 446 females) adult from Santal habitat villages were measured. Commonly used indicators i.e., weight, height and BMI, are used to evaluate nutritional status. Significant ge-group difference both in males (F = 16.164, p < 0.001) and females (F = 8.213, p < 0.001) were recorded. Significant sex differences in mean BMI were observed in age range 18-39 years (t = 8.243, p < 0.001), age range 40-55 years (t = 2.899, p < 0.05) and age range > 55 years as (t = 2.242, p < 0.05). The females were highly energy deficient than their male counterpart; females have CED (Gd-III = 13.7, Gd-II = 16.1, Gd-I = 30.9) then males (Gd-III = 6.7, Gd-II = 6.4, Gd-I = 19.4). There was a highly significant difference between sexes in CED prevalence (x^2= 64.977; df = 4; p < 0.001). BMI was highly negatively significantly correlated with age and age^2. Sex had significant (F= 71.394, p< 0.001) effect on BMI. Even after controlling for age, sex explained 8.1% of variation in BMI. Santal adults of Purulia, India are in very critical situation for all age groups and the women and oldest among them were experiencing the most critical situation with respect to their health and nutritional status.

Keywords: Santals; India; Body mass index; Chronic energy deficiency.

INTRODUCTION

Body Mass index is a measure of the body weight relative to height that is accociated with body fat and health risk. It was developed in the mid 1800's by a Belgian mathematician named Adolphe Quetelet. It is equal to the weight, divided by the square of the height. Anthropometric measurements play a very important role in the assessment of nutrition in human population. Quetlet or body mass index (BMI) is widely accepted as one of the best indicators of nutritional status for the adults [1-3]. It is also suggested that the BMI may effects more nutritionally than genetically related changes [4], despite wide variation between human populations in weight and height [5, 6]. A BMI < 18.5 kg/m2 is widely used as a practical measure of chronic energy or hunger deficiency (CED), i.e., a 'steady' underweight in which an individual is in energy balance irrespective of a loss in body weight or body energy stores [7]. Thus the use of BMI as an anthropometric indicator of nutritional status may be more appropriate in a country with diverse ethnic groups like India [8]. The assessment is done by observing the deviations of the anthropometric measures from the normal standard. The basic causes of undernutrition in developing countries are poverty, poor hygienic conditions and little access to preventive and health care [9, 10]. In developing countries like India, anthropometry, despite its inherent limitations, remains the most practical tool for assessing the nutritional status of the community [11].

India is a land of numerous culture and people. The different forms of people found here out numbers any country [12]. Indian tribal people amount to an 8.14 percentage of the total population of the country, numbering 84.51 million, according to the 2001 census. These tribal people reside in approximately 15 percent of the country's area. Indian tribals primarily reside in various ecological and geo-climatical conditions ranging from plains, forests, hills and inaccessible areas, that perhaps lies dotted in the panoramic Indian terrain. According to article-342 of the Indian Constitution, at present, there exist 697 tribes notified by the Central Government. These Indian tribal groups have been notified to reside in more than one State. More than half of the Indian tribal population is concentrated in the States of Madhya Pradesh, Chhatisgarh, Maharastra, Orissa, Jharkhand and Gujarat [13]. It is due to the presence of these tribes that our country has received its varied flavour. West Bengal is a state in the eastern region of India and is the nation's fourth most populous [14]. It is also the seventh most populous sub-national entity in the world [14]. Till now, data are scanty on the anthropometric and nutritional status of various tribal populations of India [15-21]. It has been recently suggested [16] that there is urgent need to evaluate the nutritional status of various tribes of India. The objective of the present study is evaluate the nutritional status of the adult Santals of Purulia and to compare the findings with the existing published work on the nutritional status (assessed by BMI) of adult tribal populations of West Bengal.

MATERIALS AND METHODS

This chapter was community based, cross-sectional study conducted in Santal villages of Purulia District, that are situated about 250 km from Kolkata, the capital of West Bengal, India. This study was carried out from December, 2009 to January 2010. A total of 791 (345 males and 446 females) above 18 years were measured. Data were collected after obtaining the necessary approval from the villagers; participants were informed about the objectives before the commencement of measurements. Information on age, gender, weight and height were collected on a pre-tested questionnaire by house-to house visit following interview and examination. Height and weight measurements were taken on each subject by the first author following the standard techniques [22].

According to the 2001 census, the district contains population of 2,536,516 of whom 1,298,078 are males and 1,238,438 are females out of whom 19.35% are Scheduled Castes and 19.22% are Scheduled Tribes. Purulia district is having second highest percentage of tribal population (18.3%) after Jalpaiguri (18.9%) in West Bengal. Some of the major tribes of Purulia district are Santals, Bhumijs, Kherias and Shabars. Among them, Santals consist of the highest population concentration in Purulia. According to the report of West Bengal Scheduled Castes and Tribes Facts and Information, Special Series No. 32, 1989, Santals, among all the tribal communities of Purulia district, comprise 62.66%. Tribal societies of Purulia are having distinct characteristics, where most of them are of Proto-Australoids groups with dark skin colour, sunken nose and lower forehead. As far as linguistic affiliation is concerned the languages spoken by the tribes in Purulia district are mostly from Austro-Asiatic family where people belonging to Munda branch speak Santhali, Gondi, and Kheria. Purulia district, a part of the Chhotanagpur Plateau in India constitutes an area of particularly low agricultural productivity and a high incidence and severity of poverty. Moreover, the incidence of poverty among rural households in the Chhotanagpur Plateau is estimated to be among the highest in Asia. The district of Purulia is the westernmost district of West Bengal, girdled by the Tropic of Cancer, and its latitudinal and longitudinal extents are from 22°42′35″ to 23°42′00″North and from 85°49′25″ to 86°54′37″East respectively. Purulia has its boundaries on the east with Paschim Medinipur and Bankura districts of West Bengal; on the north with Bardhaman district of West Bengal; on the north- west, west and south- west with Jharkhand state. The total geographical area of the district is 6259 sq. kms (Census 2001), out of which the urban and rural areas consist of 79.37 sq. kms (1.27%) (Municipalities & Non-Municipalities) and 6179.63 sq. kms (98.73%), respectively.

The BMI was computed using the following standard equation: BMI = Weight (kg) / height (m^2). Nutritional status was evaluated using internationally accepted BMI guidelines [23]. The following cut-off points were used:

CED BMI <18.5
Normal: BMI = 18.5-24.9
Overweight: BMI ≥ 25.0
CED was further divided into CED III, CED II and CED I as BMI < 16.0, 16.0-16.9 and 17.0-18.4 kg/m^2, respectively.

We followed the World Health Organization's classification (1995) of the public health problem of low BMI, based on adult populations worldwide. This classification categorises prevalence according to percentage of a population with BMI< 18.5.

Low (5-9%): warning sign, monitoring required.
Medium (10-19%): poor situation.
High (20-39%): serious situation.
Very high (≥ 40%): critical situation.

Student's t-tests were performed to test for sex differences in mean BMI between sexes. Age-group difference was performed by ANOVA. Sex differences in CED were determined by chi-square test. Impact of age & age^2 on BMI were determined by bivariate correlation (r). Multiple linear regression analyses were performed to determine the impact of sex on BMI after controlling age. All statistical analyses were undertaken using the SPSS Statistical Package. Statistical significance was set at $p < 0.05$.

RESULTS

The mean & standard deviation of age among males and females were 39.12 years (16.78) and 37.21 years (15.46). Thus both sexes had almost similar mean ages. Table 1 presents the mean weight, height and BMI of the study subjects. The age group statistics (mean ± standard deviation) of derived index (Body Mass Index) and their comparative statements between the sexes (measured by Student t test) and age-group difference (measured by ANOVA test) were presented in table 2. The mean (± standard deviation) age (Range 18-39 years) of the males were $19.91 kg/m^2$ (2.45), (Range 40-55 years) is $19.59 \ kg/m^2$ (2.22) and (> 55 years) is $18.11 \ kg/m^2$ (2.07). Similarly, mean (± standard deviation) age (Range 18-39 years) of the females are $18.28 \ kg/m^2$ (1.89), (Range 40-55 years) is $18.52 \ kg/m^2$ (2.49) and (> 55 years) is $17.28 \ kg/m^2$ (2.43). Table 2 also shows the significant age-group difference both in males (F = 16.164, $p < 0.001$) and females (F = 16.164, $p < 0.001$). Significant sex differences in mean BMI were observed in age range 18-39 years (t = 8.243, $p < 0.001$), age range 40-55 years (t = 2.899, $p < 0.05$) and age range > 55 years as (t = 2.242, $p < 0.05$). Table 3 shows the prevalence of CED (among males and females) of the Santals of Purulia, West Bengal, is shown in Table 3. From this table it can be inferred that, in general, the females were highly energy deficient than their male counterpart; females have CED (Gd-III = 13.7, Gd-II = 16.1, Gd-I = 30.9) then males (Gd-III = 6.7, Gd-II = 6.4, Gd-I = 19.4). There was a highly significant difference between sexes in CED prevalence (x^2= 64.977; df = 4; $p < 0.001$).

Prevalence of CED among men (Table 4) based on BMI clearly revealed that with the advancement of age prevalence of CED also inclined from 18-39 years to > 55 years gradually and the prevalence of CED increase was maximum (16.0 %, based on BMI) for >55 years. Similarly prevalence of

Table 1. Mean (sd) anthropometric characteristics of the subjects

Variable	Men (n = 345)	Women (n = 446)	t
Weight (kg)	49.37 (7.85)	39.68 (5.83)	19.90***
Height (cm)	158.98 (6.52)	147.65 (5.69)	26.05***
BMI (kg/m^2)	19.46 (2.43)	18.10 (2.15)	8.00***

Standard deviations are presented in parentheses.
***p < 0.001

Table 2. Age trends in mean BMI among the subjects

Sex	Mean (SD)			F	p
	18-39 years	40-55 years	> 55 years		
Men	19.91 (2.45)	19.59 (2.22)	18.11 (2.07)	16.164	0.001
Women	18.28 (1.89)	18.52 (2.49)	17.28 (2.43)	8.213	0.001
T	8.243 ***	2.899*	2.242*		

t = Sex difference in each age group:
* p < 0.05
***p < 0.001.

Table 3. Nutritional status of the subjects based on BMI

Nutritional Status	BMI (kg/m^2)	Men	Women
CED III	<16.0	6.7	13.7
CED II	16.0 -16.9	6.4	16.1
CED I	17.0 – 18.4	19.4	30.9
Total CED	Upto 18.4	32.5	60.8
Normal	18.5 -24.9	65.5	38.3
Overweight	25.0 – 29.9	2.0	0.9

All figures presented are percentages.
Sex difference: chi-square = 64.977, p < 0.001.

CED among women based on BMI showed gradual inclined in CED from 18-30 years to 55 years and the maximum increase was observed as 10.0 % for 55 years women.

BMI was highly negatively significantly correlated with age and age^2. With the increase in age, BMI decreased in both sexes (male r = -0.227**; female r = -0.158*). Similar findings with age^2 (male r = -0.256**; female r = -0.180*) were observed. The sex combined correlation with age and age^2 were -0.167** & -0.191**, respectively. Multiple linear regression analyses of BMI (dependent variable) with age and sex revealed that both these independent

Table 4. Age group wise nutritional status of the subjects based on BMI

Nutritional status	Men			Women		
	18-39 years (n=197)	40-55 years (n=75)	> 55 years (n=73)	18-39 years (n=280)	40-55 years (n=91)	> 55 years (n=75)
CED (< 18.50)	23.9	36.0	52.1	58.9	59.3	69.3
Normal (18.50-24.99)	72.6	64.0	47.9	40.7	37.4	30.7
Overweight (> 25.0)	3.6	0.0	0.0	0.4	3.3	0.0

All figures presented are percentages.
Sex difference: chi-square =64.977, df =4, p < 0.001.

variables had significant negative effect (results not presented) on BMI. The effect of sex (t = -8.450, p < 0.001) was more than that of age (t = -5.468, p < 0.001). Sex had significant (F= 71.394, p< 0.001) effect on BMI. Even after controlling for age, sex explained 8.1% of variation in BMI.

Thus, it is clear from the tables that Santal adults of Purulia, India are in very critical situation for all age groups and the women and oldest among them were experiencing the most critical situation with respect to their health and nutritional status.

DISCUSSION

Comparisons of mean BMI (among males and females) of the present study with various tribal population of India are shown in Table 5. From this table it is clear that Santal (20.5 kg/m^2) males of West Bengal [24] have the highest mean BMI and Warli (16.8 kg/m^2) males of Maharastra [25] have the lowest mean BMI. Similarly, Jarwa females (19.8 kg/m^2) [26] have the highest and Muda females (17.7 kg/m^2) [27] of West Bengal have the least mean BMI out of all the studied tribal population shown in table 5.

In general, prevalence of CED is presented in Figure 1 (a-g), overall CED was highest in Maharastra (59.6 %), who experience the most critical situation out of the total studied tribal population (available reports, Figure 1) of India followed by Jharkhand (58.8 %), Tamil Nadu (55.0 %), Orissa (49.5 %), Kerala (37.8 %), Andaman & Nicobar Island (29.5 %) and Assam &

Table 5. Comparison of mean BMI among tribal population of Inda

State	Population	Male BMI (kg/m^2) Mean	Female BMI (kg/m^2) Mean	Overall	Reference
West Bengal	Bhumij	18.7	18.4	18.6	Ghosh, 2007
	Dhimal	19.5	19.1	19.3	Banik et al, 2007
	Kora Mudi	18.7	18.3	18.5	Bose et al, 2006b
	Kora Mudi	18.6	18.3	18.5	Bisai et al, 2008
	Lodha	19.5	19.3	19.4	Mondal, 2007
	Munda	18.7	17.7	18.2	Ghosh & Bharati, 2006
	Oraon	18.8	19.7	19.3	Mittal & Sivastava, 2006
	Santal	20.0	19.3	19.7	Bose et al, 2006c
	Santal	18.5	18.7	18.6	Ghosh & Mallik, 2007
	Santal	20.5	19.5	20.0	Mukhopadhyay, 2009
	Lodha	19.5	--	--	Bose et al, 2008
	Bhumij	18.7	--	--	Bose et al, 2008
Orissa	Bathudi	18.4	--	--	Bose & Chakrabarty, 2005
	Bhuiya	19.4	--	--	Chakraborty et al, 2008
	Gond	18.1	--	--	Chakraborty et al, 2008
	Khond	19.2	--	--	Chakraborty et al, 2008
	Munda	19.1	--	--	Chakraborty et al, 2008
	Paroja	17.3	--	--	Chakraborty et al, 2008
	Santal	18.3	--	--	Chakraborty et al, 2008
	Savara	18.5	--	--	Chakraborty et al, 2008
	Santal	19.6	--	--	Bose et al, 2006
Jharkhand	Oraon	18.5	--	--	Datta Banik , 2008
	Oraon	18.0	--	--	Chakraborty & Bose, 2008

State	Population	Male BMI (kg/m2) Mean	Female BMI (kg/m2) Mean	Overall	Reference
Maharastra	Andh	17.1	--	--	Adak et al, 2006
	Bhil	18.0	--	--	Adak et al, 2006
	Gond	18.3	--	--	Adak et al, 2006
	Kathodi	17.0	--	--	Adak et al, 2006
	Korku	18.3	--	--	Adak et al, 2006
	Mahadeokoli	18.2	--	--	Adak et al, 2006
	Warli	16.8	--	--	Adak et al, 2006
	Kol	18.8	--	--	Rajesh et al,
	Manjhi	19.4	--	--	Rajesh et al,
	Sonr	17.6	--	--	Rajesh et al,
	Korwa	20.8	--	--	Rajesh et al,
	Sahariya	18.1	--	--	Rajesh et al,
Kerala	Mannan	20.2	19.1	19.7	John & Ramadas, 200
Andaman & Nicobar Island	Jarwa	18.9	19.8	19.4	Sahani, 2003
	Onge	--	--	21.0	Rao et al, 2005
Assam	Boro-Kacharis	19.8	--	--	Khongsdier, 2001
	Lalung	19.2	--	--	Khongsdier, 2001
	Mechs	20.5	--	--	Khongsdier, 2001
	Miris	19.6	--	--	Khongsdier, 2001
Meghalaya	Phars	19.9	--	--	Khongsdier, 2001
West Bengal	Santal	19.46	18.10	18.8	Present study

Meghalaya (20 %). Among the tribals Kathodi (90.0 %) from Maharastra have the most critical situation and Mechs (20.0 %) of Assam have the least CED prevalence out of the 51 studied tribals from different States of India.

Santal males and females of present study have mean BMI of (19.5 kg/m^2 & 18.1 kg/m^2) and BMI of the tribals males and females of West Bengal (combined all the studied tribals of West Bengal) was (19.2 kg/m^2 & 18.8 kg/m^2) and there were no significant difference with the mean BMI with state. BMI of the tribes of West Bengal was in the range of 18.5-20.5 kg/m^2. Moreover, the rate of CED among Santal of our study was 46.7 % while CED rates varied between 31.6 % and 58.5 %. These rates were in the category high (20-39%) to very high ($\geq$40%). These results clearly indicated that, Santals of present study were under serious to critical nutritional stress.

 Subal Das and Kaushik Bose

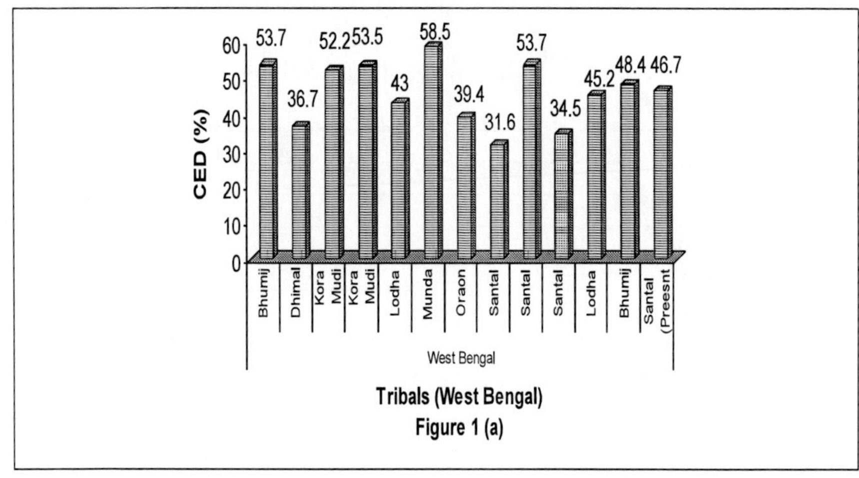

Tribals (West Bengal)
Figure 1 (a)

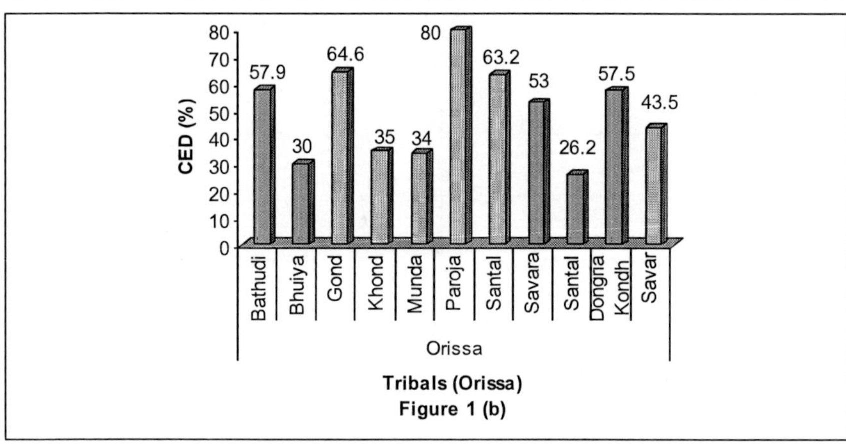

Tribals (Orissa)
Figure 1 (b)

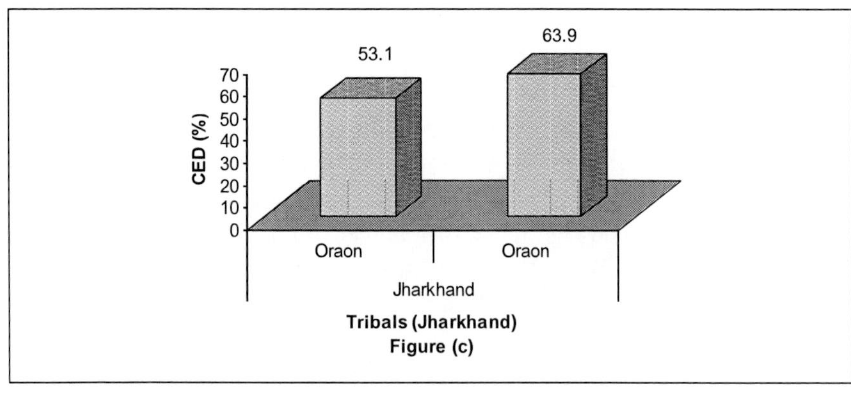

Tribals (Jharkhand)
Figure (c)

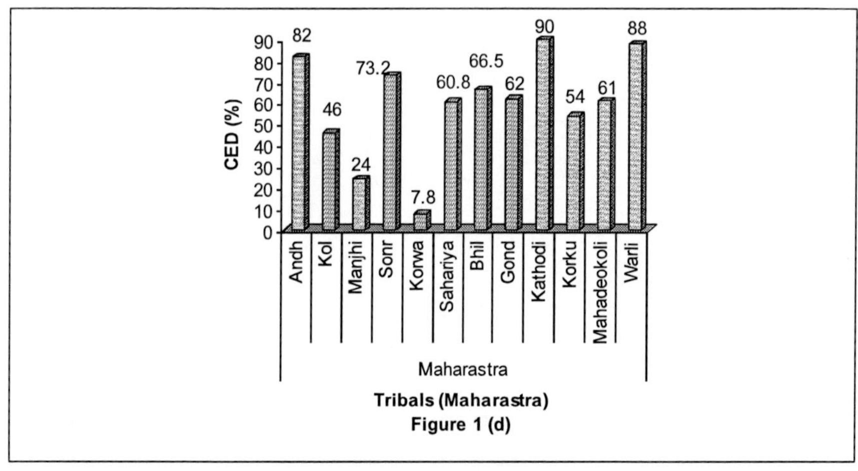

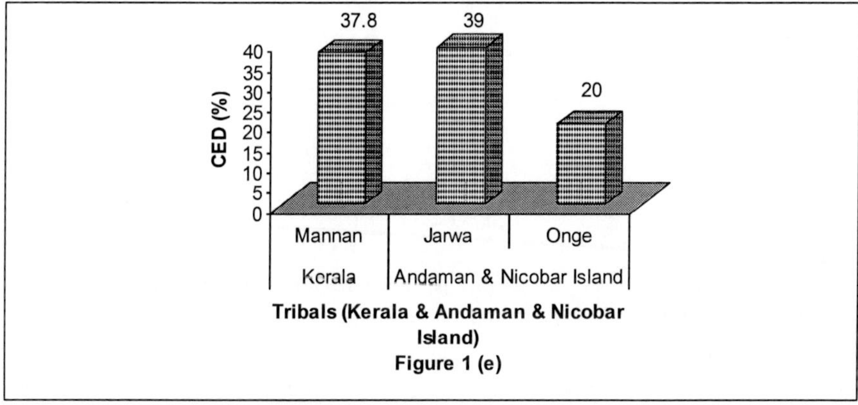

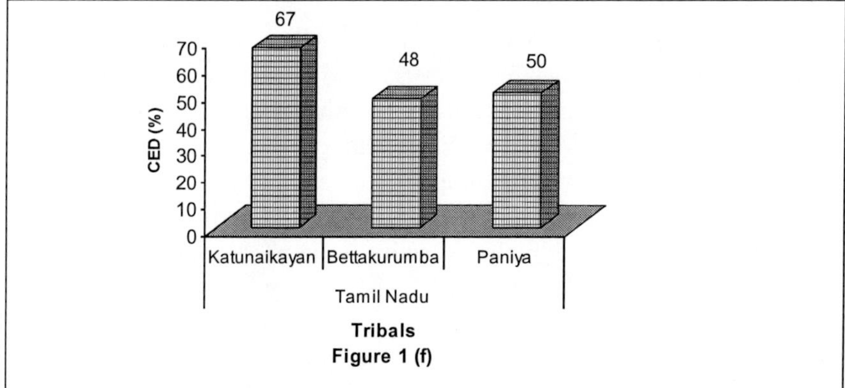

Figure 1. (continued).

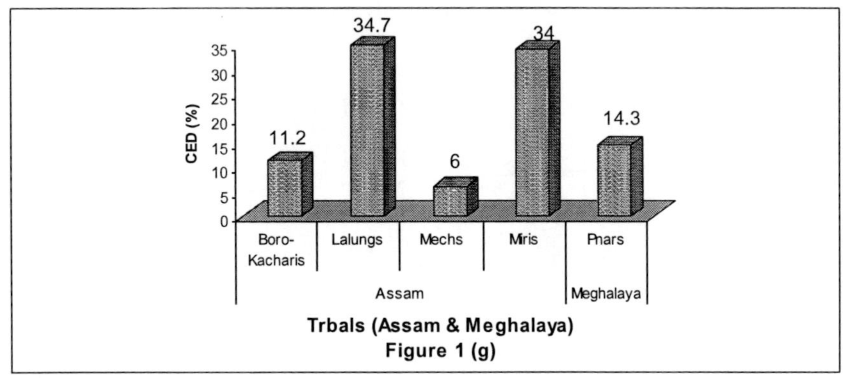

Figures 1(a-g). Comparison of CED prevalence among tribal populations of India.

According to National Family Health Statistics- 3 report [28], the prevalence of undernutrition in India is 33.0% among males and 28.1% among females. In urban areas, these figures were 19.8% and 17.5%, respectively. In rural areas these were 38.8% and 33.1%, respectively. However, the situation is much worse in West Bengal with corresponding prevalence of 37.7% and 31.6%, respectively. Among urban males and females they were 19.9% and 15.5%, respectively. The corresponding rural figures were 44.9% (males) and 38.0% (females).

The study done by Adak et. al., [25] shows that the prevalence of CED among the tribals of Maharastra was highest Kathudi (90.0 %), but it should be kept in mind that the sample size of the studied tribals from Maharastra were very small (n=50) and with the increase of sample size (n=100 or 200) the prevalence of CED also declines. Several recent studies from India [29, 30, 26, 16, 17] have utilized BMI to study nutritional status of tribal populations. Therefore, the use of BMI and WHO (1995) BMI based cut-off points for the evaluation of CED are valid for use among tribal populations of India. The primary importance, from the public health perspective is the need for immediate nutritional intervention programs to be implemented among Santals of Purulia and all other tribal groups experiencing nutritional stress. The Indian Government should play an active role in reducing the rates of undernutrition among tribal people. Although priority must be given to tribal groups having the highest rates of undernutrition, all groups must be incorporated in these food supplementation programs. It is imperative that the recommendations should include not only adequate dietary intake but also various ways in which they can enhance their socio-economic status through improved education and employment opportunities. It is expected that better educational attainment will lead to more scope for employment and healthier dietary practices. It is here that relevant government authorities should play a proactive role in reducing the rates of undernutrition among tribals. It has already been emphasized that there exists variation in social and economic conditions among tribes of India [31]. This variation must be taken into account before tribal-specific intervention programmes are formulated and initiated. Lastly, since nutritional status is intricately linked with dietary habits as well as the ecology of the population, further research should be undertaken to investigate, in details, these factors. Each tribal population has its unique food habits [32]. Moreover, there are distinct inter-tribal differences in the environment in which they reside, i.e. ecology of the population [32]. The studies reviewed here did not deal with these factors as they were beyond the scope of study. These are limitations which must be addressed in future studies. Therefore, it is imperative that future studies on tribal populations include these parameters when investigating their nutritional status. Similar studies should also be undertaken among other tribal populations in India since they constitute a sizeable portion of India's population. Moreover, since undernutrition has several underlying causes [23, 33] future investigations should aim at identifying the likely cause(s) of high rates of undernutrition among Indian tribal populations.

CONCLUSION

From this chapter it can be concluded that the nutritional status of Santals was critical; females and oldest peoples experiencing the most critical situation then the others. This further indicates reduction of mean BMI with increasing age. As well as those cited by us, provided strong evidence that, in general, Santals and other tribal populations of India were experiencing serious to critical nutritional stress.

ACKNOWLEDGMENTS

The authors express there thanks to the tribals for their cooperation. Financial assistance in the form of Senior Research Fellowship (SRF) to the first author (SD) from University Grants Commission, Government of India (UGC- ref. no. 223/NET- Dec. 2008).

REFERENCES

[1] James, W.P.T., Ferro-Luzzi, A., & Waterlow, J.C. (1988). Definition of chronic energy deficiency in adults. *Eur J Clin Nutr,* 42:969-981.

[2] Ferro-Luzzi, *A.,* Sette, S., Franklin, M., James, T.P.W. (1992). "A simplified approach of assessing adult chronic deficiency". *European Journal of Clinical Nutrition,* 46, 173-186.

[3] Shetty, P.S., & James, W.P.T. (1994). Report of the Food and Agricultural Organization: Body Mass Index: A measure of Chronic Energy Deficiency in Adults. *Food and Nutrition*, Paper No. 56. Rome.

[4] Rolland-Cachera, M.F. (1993). "Body composition during adolescence: Methods, Limitations, and determinants." *Hormone Research*, 39 (Suppl 3): 25- 40.

[5] Eveleth, P.B., & Tanner, J.M. (1990). *Worldwide Variation in Human Growth*, 2nd edn (Cambridge: Cambridge University Press).

[6] Majumder, P. P., Shanker, B.U., Basu, A., Malhotra, K.C., Gupta, R., Mukhopadhyay, B., Viyayakumar, M., & Roy, S.K. (1990). Anthropometric variation in India: a statistical appraisal. *Current Anthropology*, 31, 94-103.

[7] Khongsdier, R. (2005). "BMI and morbidity in relation to body composition: a crosssectional study of a rural community in North-East India." *British Journal of Nutrition,* 93, 101-107.

[8] Khongsdier, R. (2001). Body mass index of adult males in 12 populations of Northeast India. *Annals of Human Biology*, VOL. 28, NO. 4, 374-383.

[9] Mitra, A., (1985). The nutrition situation in India. In *Nutrition and Development*, edited by M. Biswas and P. Andersen (Oxford: Oxford University Press), pp. 142-162.

[10] World Health Organization. (1990). Diet, nutrition and the prevention of chronic disease. *WHO Technical Report Series No. 797* (Geneva: World Health Organization).

[11] Ghosh, A., Bose, K., & Das Chaudhuri, A.B. (2001). Age and sex variations in adiposity and central fat distribution among elderly Bengalee Hindus of Calcutta, India. *Annals of Human Biology,* 28: 616–623.

[12] *http://en.wikipedia.org/wiki/List_of_Scheduled_Tribes_in_India. Retrieved April 18, 2011* at 7.30 PM.

[13] *http://www.indianetzone.com/37/indian_tribes.htm.* Retrieved April 19, 2011 at 1.10 PM.

[14] *"India: Administrative Divisions (population and area)". Census of India.* *http://www.world* gazetteer.com/wg.php?x=&men=gadm&lng=en&des=wg&geo =104&srt=npan&col=abcdefghinoq&msz=1500&va=x. Retrieved April 17, 2009.

[15] Arlappa, N., Balakrishna, N., Brahmam, G.N., & Vijayaraghavan, K. (2005). "Nutritional status of the tribal elderly in India." *Journal of Nutrition for the Elderly*, 25: 23-39.

[16] Bose, K., & Chakraborty, F. (2005). "Anthropometric characteristics and nutritional Status based on body mass index of adult Bathudis: a tribal population of Keonjhar District, Orissa, India." *Asia Pacific Journal of Clinical Nutrition,* 14, 80-82.

[17] Bose, K., Chakraborty, F., Bisai, S., Khatun, A., & Bauri, H. (2006a). "Body mass index and nutritional status of adult Savar tribals of Keonjhar District, Orissa, India." *Asia Pacific Journal of Public Health,* 18, 3-7.

[18] Bose, K., Ganguli, S., Mamtaz, H., Mukhopadhyay, A., & Bhadra, M. (2006b). "High prevalence of undernutrition among adult Kora Mudi tribals of Bankura District, West Bengal, India". *Anthropological Science,* 114, 65-68.

[19] Bose, K., Banerjee, S., Bisai, S., Mukhopadhyay, A., & Bhadra, M. (2006c). "Anthropometric profile and chronic energy deficiency among adult Santal tribals of Jhargram, West Bengal, India: Comparison with other tribal populations of Eastern India." *Ecology of Food and Nutrition,* 45, I-II.

[20] Bose, K., Bisai, S., & Chakraborty, F., (2006d). "Age variations in anthropometric and body composition characteristics and underweight among male Bathudisa tribal population of Keonjhar District, Orissa, India." *Collegium Antropologicum*, 30, 771-775.

[21] Ghosh, A., & Bala, K.S. (2006). "Anthropometric characteristics and nutritional status of Kondh: a tribal population of Kandhmal District, Orissa, India." *Annals of Human Biology,* 33, 641-647.

[22] Lohman, T.G., Roche, A.F., & Martorell, R. (1988). *Anthropometric Standardization Reference Manual.* Chicago: Human Kinetics Books.

[23] World Health Organization. (1995). *Physical Status: the Use and Interpretation of Anthropometry.* Technical Report Series no. 854. Geneva: World Health Organization.

[24] Mukhopadhyay, A. (2009). Anthropometric characteristics and undernutrition among adult Santal tribe of Birbhum District, West Bengal, India. *Anthropological Science.* 1-4.

[25] Adak, D.K, Gautam, R.K, Gharami, A.K. (2006). Assessment of Nutritional Status Through Body Mass Index among adult males of 7 tribal population of Maharashtra, India. *Mal. J. Nutr.* Vol.12 (1). pp 23-31.

[26] Sahani, R. (2003). "Nutritional and health status of the Jarawas: A preliminary report." *Journal of Anthropological Survey of India,* 52, 47-65.

[27] Ghosh, R., & Bharati, P. (2006). "Nutritional status of adults among Munda and Pod populations in a peri urban area of Kolkata City, India." *Asia Pacific Journal of Public Health,* 18 (2), 12-20.

[28] National Family Health Survey (NFHS-3). (2005-2006). *Report on West Bengal by International Institute for Population Science (IIPS),* India, Volume II, Mumbai, IIPS.

[29] Yadav, Y.S., Singh, P., & Kumar, A. (1999). "Nutritional status of tribals and non-tribals in Bihar." *Indian Journal of Preventive and Social Medicine,* 30, 101-106.

[30] Gogoi, G. & Sengupta, S. (2002). "Body mass index among the Dibongiya Deoris of Assam, India." *Journal of Human Ecology,* 13, 271-273.

[31] Topal, Y.S., & Samal, P.K. (2001). Causes for variation in social and economic conditions among tribes of Indian Central Himalaya: A comparative study. *Man in India.* 81: 87-88.

[32] Mandal, H., Mukherjee, S., & Datta, A. (2002). *India– An Illustrated Atlas of Tribal World. Kolkata: Anthropological Survey of India.*

[33] Lee, R.D. & Nieman, D.C. (2003). *Nutritional Assessment.* New York: McGraw Hill.

In: New Trends in Body Mass Index Research   ISBN 978-1-61942-430-2
Editors: A. Vermeulen and E. De Smet   © 2012 Nova Science Publishers, Inc.

Chapter V

BODY MASS INDEX AND FAT DISTRIBUTION CIRCUMPOLAR PEOPLES: IMPLICATIONS FOR THE MEASUREMENT OF OBESITY AND FOR THE OPTIMIZATION OF LIFESTYLE

Roy J. Shephard[*]
Faculty of Physical Education and Health,
University of Toronto, Toronto, ON, Canada

ABSTRACT

Information on the body size and distribution of body fat in circumpolar populations is of particular interest when examining the validity of simple methods of estimating the overall body fat content; use of the body mass index (BMI) is complicated by the atypical body build of the traditional Inuit and by the manner in which this historic phenotype has changed with acculturation to the lifestyle of industrialized society in recent years. Comparison of body mass index data with other measures of body fat content show that the former can give a misleading impression of obesity in populations with a short stature and/or a muscular body build. Over the past four de cades, the "natural experiment" of acculturation to southern Canadian patterns of diet isnd physical activity has led to rapid changes of physique among arctic populations, including a deterioration of physical fitness and a substantial increase of average

---

[*] Phone: 604-898-5527 Fax: 604-898-5724 E-mail: royjshep@shaw.ca.

body fat content. Skinfold readings suggest a substantial accumulation of body fat, but because of a reduction in lean tissue, this is not always reflected in the BMI. The replacement of hunting by the consumption of store-purchased food and the adoption of a sedentary lifestyle present nutritional and environmental challenges to many circumpolar populations, but poor metabolic health is not an inevitable consequence of adopting a "modern" lifestyle. As in urban, industrialized society, good health can be maintained through the deliberate incorporation of adequate physical activity into daily life.

In this chapter, we describe briefly epidemiological use of the body mass index (BMI), and consider critically its limitations as an index of body fat content in individuals and in populations with particular reference to the circumpolar environment. We next examine the physique of traditional, circumpolar peoples, and consider the impact of their unusual physical characteristics upon the BMI and the distribution of body fat as assessed from skinfold readings. We discuss changes in both the physique and the body fat content of northern peoples that have accompanied their transition from hunting to the purchase of store food and the adoption of a sedentary lifestyle, and finally consider whether the resulting adverse changes in health status are an inevitable consequence of acculturation.

EPIDEMIOLOGICAL USE OF THE BODY MASS INDEX

Epidemiologists have commonly assessed the obesity of populations resulting patterns of health in terms of the BMI, expressed in kg/m^2. A U-shaped relationship between body mass index and mortality has been recognized since the studies of Andres [1, 2]. Mortality is lowest in those with a BMI in the range 20-25 kg/m^2, and prognosis is poorer with a BMI <20 kg/m^2 or >25 kg/m^2. There is general agreement that the adverse consequences of a high BMI reflect diseases associated with an increased body fat content. However, reasons for the adverse effect of a BMI <20 kg/m^2 are less certain. Given the ability of smoking to curtail appetite, one suggestion has been that those with a low BMI died of smoking-related diseases. A second possible factor may be undetected disease such as cancer or tuberculosis.

Critics of early BMI studies have noted that the populations involved were biased (those purchasing Life Insurance in the U.S. and Canada). Also, most of the height and weight data were self-reported, with a resultant risk of under-reporting actual body mass [3]. Moreover, it has been argued that even at the high end of the BMI curve, the adverse effect of obesity may have been under-estimated because smokers and individuals with pre-existing neoplastic disease skewed the entire U-curve in a leftward direction. However, a recent analysis of BMI data from a large prospective cancer study carefully excluded pre-existing disease and calculated a separate curve for smokers [4]. This study confirmed earlier reports. It showed a significantly poorer prognosis among North American adults who were overweight (a body mass index in the range 25.0-29.9 kg/m^2), with a further deterioration in those who were clinically obese (>30 kg/m^2). Further, the prognosis was poorer for both smokers and non-smokers with a BMI <20 kg/m.^{2} Possibly, a low BMI reflects a lack of physical activity and thus a paucity of lean tissue, exposing the individual concerned to all of the health problems associated with a lack of physical fitness [5].

CRITIQUE OF THE BODY MASS INDEX

Although the BMI has proven a useful empirical tool in many large scale epidemiological surveys, there are several inherent problems in using this index as a surrogate of body fat content, particularly when it is applied to smaller or selected populations. Some investigators have argued on mechanical, hydrodynamic and thermal grounds that there should be a cubic rather than a quadratic relationship between body mass and height [6]. This is far from an academic question. For instance, one sample of children in Guam had a very short average stature; a cubic ratio would have classed them as having a normal body build, but use of either a simple or a quadratic ratio would have suggested that they were unusually thin [7]. Even if one accepts that a quadratic relationship is the most appropriate, calculation of the BMI immediately assumes that the relationship between body mass and height^2 is linear, passing through the origin of height and body mass axes. This may not be a major problem when comparing people of similar physique, but it is an important issue when populations are of radically different body build. It is then more appropriate to determine an allometric relationship using least squares regression techniques.

The correlation between the BMI and the usually accepted gold standard of body fat content (hydrostatic weighing) is typically quite weak, unless the test sample includes individuals ranging widely in body dimensions. Thus, in one sample of some 80 Toronto schoolchildren, correlation coefficients were only 0.37 in boys and 0.51 in girls [8]. The index necessarily assumes that inter-individual differences in body mass reflect corresponding differences in body fat content. However, in a young adult the body mass may be increased not by fat, but rather by lean tissue, as a consequence of muscular training or the abuse of anabolic steroids. Likewise, the body mass of the elderly may fall below anticipated values because of a loss of muscle tissue (sarcopenia) or bone mineral (osteoporosis).

A final important limitation of the BMI is that it provides no indication as to whether the accumulation of body fat is peripheral or central in distribution, although the latter has a much greater adverse significance for health [9,10].

PHYSIQUE OF TRADITIONAL CIRCUMPOLAR POPULATIONS AND BODY MASS INDEX

At first inspection, the BMI might seem a very helpful approach to determining the body fat content of arctic populations. It is very costly to air-lift sophisticated electronic equipment to isolated settlements, and even if funding is obtained for this purpose, functioning of the equipment is hampered by a instability of electrical voltages and frequencies. Likewise, it remains far from clear that skin-fold and body impedance formulae as determined on "white" populations are appropriate when predicting the body fat content of indigenous peoples [11]. Unfortunately, the physique of traditional circumpolar peoples also differs substantially from that of the "white" populations used in defining optimal BMI values, and uncritical use of BMI has led to some erroneous diagnoses of obesity.

There is little disagreement that traditional circumpolar residents have a substantial body mass in relation to height. This characteristic was very evident in the first detailed study of the Inuit community of Igloolik that we completed in 1969-70 [12]. At this time, the Igloolik population had just moved from igloos and tents to a permanent, government-constructed settlement, and many members of the community were still active hunters, with a very high daily energy expenditure. The average body mass of adult male villagers exceeded actuarial norms by 8-10 kg. Nutrition Canada made parallel observations in many arctic villages during the early 1970s. This led them to conclude that a high proportion of Inuit were obese [13], a view probably reinforced by their round faces, short noses and bulky clothing of the villagers. However, our data for Igloolik underlined that the high BMI stood in marked contrast with average skinfold thicknesses, which were much less than in most surveys of southern Canadians. A study of the St. Lawrence Island Inuit [14] suggested that a short leg length in relation to sitting height [15, 16, 17] was responsible for the anomalously high BMI values.

It has been estimated that differences in relative leg length can modify the BMI by as much 5-10 units [18, 19]. A study of 489 Nunavik Inuit from the year 2004 [20, 21] confirmed continuing misdiagnosis of obesity from the standard interpretation of BMI values. However, studies of Siberian Yupik [14] and Greenlandic Inuit [22] indicated that although leg lengths were short, the sitting height was similar to that in white populations. Much more appropriate proportions of obese individuals were identified when the BMI data for the Nunavik were standardized in terms of sitting height [20,21]. However, there plainly remains scope for further study, using more sophisticated techniques to study both the amount and the distribution of body fat [23].

A further factor augmenting body mass in relation to height, at least in the community of Igloolik, was an above average muscle development, occasioned by the physical demands of life in a harsh environment. Evaluations of muscle force were complicated by differences in body mass and leverage relative to white immigrants living in Igloolik, although leg strength appeared to be substantially greater than that of white immigrants living in the same community [24]. This was confirmed by determinations of lean body mass, using deuterated water; values for the Inuit averaged 3.54g per meter of stature, as compared with typical values of 3.0 g/m in urban "white" males [12]. Measurements of arm muscle cross-sectional area also reported values between the 50th and 85th percentiles of U.S. norms (15).

Given these issues of short stature and muscularity, it is not surprising that the standard interpretation of body mass index values [13] led to the erroneous view that traditional Inuit were obese.

DISTRIBUTION OF BODY FAT IN TRADITIONAL INUIT

Although it seems clear that in the traditional Inuit, the layer of sub-cutaneous fat at most of the typical skinfold measurement sites is very thin, it may be rash either to infer the distribution of body fat or to estimate the percentage of body fat from these readings. Prediction equations established for those living in temperate climates may be inappropriate for those living in the far north. In terms of thermal protection, it appears that the Inuit rely more on readily modifiable clothing assemblies than a thick layer of subcutaneous fat, but it has also been suggested that because hunting trips may combine a very high daily energy expenditure (averaging 15.4 MJ/ day) with a lack of food [25], there must be substantial internal reserves of fat to sustain metabolism during prolonged expeditions. If there is indeed such a depot, its location and its relationship to health prognosis have yet to be determined.

A recent study of Greenlandic Inuit concluded that central obesity (as determined from the ratio of waist to hip circumferences) was more prevalent in this population than in a Danish reference group (58.1% vs.17.8% of the women, and 15.9% vs. 8.3% of the men, 26). However, the central obesity appeared to carry fewer adverse health consequences than in the Danish population [27]. Lifestyle or body build factors seem to be implicated, since the metabolic health of Inuit with an apparently comparable degree of obesity was poorer among those who had emigrated to Denmark [28].

SECULAR CHANGES IN INUIT PHYSIQUE

Cross-sectional comparisons between arctic communities at various stages in the process of acculturation, together with longitudinal study of the Inuit community of Igloolik has allowed documentation of the changes in physique associated with adjustments to a modern, urbanized lifestyle. Probably because of a shift from "country" to supermarket foods (with an associated increase in the consumption of refined carbohydrates), there has been a rapid secular trend to an increase in height [29, 30]. Historically, Inuit children were short relative to cross-sectional norms of growth for those living in the urban United States [16, 29, 31]; young adults were thus short; moreover, there was an unusually rapid decrease of stature over adult life (20 mm/decade of life in active hunters, 4 mm/decade in non-hunters), apparently related to a combination of vitamin D lack and the impact of long snowmobile trips on the spine [32].

Data collected in Cumberland Sound suggest that the stature of Inuit children increased substantially between 1939 and 1968 [29], and data from Wainwright showed parallel differences between 1968 and 1977 [33]. Our observations in Igloolik cover the period from 1969-70 to 1989-90; over this time, the average height of pre-pubertal 10-year old children has increased by a further 6 mm, to the point where international growth norms are now being approached and the secular trend to taller children is disappearing. A similar trend to greater height has been observed in some young adult Inuit populations; thus, values for 16-18-year old Labrador Inuit showed an increase of 7-8 mm/decade between 1939 and 1993 [34], those for Inari Lapps increased by 50 mm and those for Skolt Lapps by 106 mm over 40 years, between 1934 and 1974 [35]. However, analyses of changes in older adults have been complicated by the "snowmobile effect," discussed above.

Studies of "white" populations in England and in the Netherlands suggest that the secular trend to greater standing height is due largely to growth of the legs [36, 37]. Assuming that the Inuit have followed a similar pattern, one would anticipate a progressive normalization of the sitting/standing height ratio and thus of the BMI. Certainly, our data for Igloolik in the period 1989/90 show a substantially normal sitting/standing height ratio [38].

In addition to becoming taller, the Igloolik population has shown a considerable decrease in strength, presumably with an associated decrease in muscle mass, over the period from 1969-70 to 1989-90. In young men, leg extension scores decreased by 37% over these two decades, and in the oldest men the loss was 45%; losses in female subjects were even larger [39]. Both the increase in height and the decrease in lean tissue inevitably influence the interpretation of changes in BMI over the corresponding period of acculturation.

SECULAR CHANGES IN BODY MASS INDEX AND SKINFOLD READINGS OF NORTHERN PEOPLES

In keeping with findings from a number of circumpolar communities, data from Igloolik showed a substantial increase of body mass index in older adults between 1969-70 and 1989-90 (for instance, in men aged 50-59 years, from 25.8 to 27.1 kg/m^2, and women of similar age from 27.5 to 31.7 kg/m^2)[40]. This was thought due to an increase of body fat content, since there was a parallel increase in the thickness of skin-folds (from an average of 7.9 mm to 15.7 mm in the males, and from 19,0 to 34.8 mm in the females of this age group). The skin-fold readings increased in similar fashion among younger adults, but in this age group the BMI had shown little increase, suggesting that an accumulation of fat had been masked by a substantial loss of lean tissue. Moreover, involvement in hunting activity (which had been associated with substantially below population average values for BMI and skinfold thickness in 1969-70) no longer showed this differential in 1989/90 [39].

Other reports on Inuit from the Keewatin region [41, 42] and Nouveau Québec [43] have further substantiated the adverse impact of acculturation upon BMI and skinfold readings. Reasons for the increase of body fat include the transition from "country" food such as arctic char with a high content of omega-3 fatty acids [44] to store food rich in salt and refined carbohydrate, a dramatic decline in the physical demands of life in northern settlements, and in young women a curtailment of lactation from several years to a few months. Because of the concentration of the population in larger settlements, there is no longer sufficient game for traditional hunting; dog teams and hand paddled vessels (umiaks) have largely disappeared, and any journeys that are made use snowmobiles, all-terrain vehicles or power boats [24].

CONSEQUENCES OF INCREASED BODY FAT FOR THE HEALTH OF NORTHERN PEOPLES

By analogy with "white" populations, an increase of body fat in northern populations should carry an increased risk of various chronic conditions, particularly cardiovascular disease, type II diabetes mellitus, and various forms of cancer. However, unlike indigenous groups in Southern Canada, in the Inuit HDL cholesterol levels have been higher and triglyceride concentrations lower than would be predicted from BMI values [45], and high BMI readings have shown little correlation with blood glucose or insulin levels [46].

It remains unclear how far this anomaly arises because the standard BMI still does not provide a reliable indication of obesity in the Inuit, and how far there may be some protection against the adverse effects of fat storage in the Inuit [47]. Correlations seem likely to become stronger as their body build comes closer to that of "white" Canadians. Given the long time course of the diseases in question, the adverse effects of obesity upon health will for some years be most evident in indigenous communities living at lower latitudes, where the process of acculturation is further advanced [48-51].

THE WAY FORWARD

Although many indigenous people still long for a return to their traditional lifestyle, this is generally precluded by increased population numbers and world-wide exploitation of natural resources. The northern peoples may be at increased risk of obesity and diabetes, because they have not previously faced the challenges of a western diet and a sedentary life. However, a deterioration in metabolic health is not inevitable. The prevention of obesity depends, as in the "white" population, on the moderation of food intake and on the voluntary incorporation of a minimum physical activity into normal daily life. In Igloolik, fitness and lifestyle programs have been initiated in the high-school gymnasium, and participants in this initiative are avoiding the deterioration of physique and accumulation of fat seen in their peers [52]. As in modern industrialized society, good health is possible if an appropriate lifestyle is adopted.

REFERENCES

[1]   Society of Actuaries. *Build Study*, 1979. Chicago: Society of Actuaries, 1979.

[2]   Andres, R. Discussion: Assessment of health status. In: Bouchard, C., Shephard, R.J., Stephens, T. et al. *Exercise, Fitness and Health*. Champaign, IL: Human Kinetics, 1990, pp. 133-136.

[3]   Stunkard AJ, Albaum JM. The accuracy of self-reported weights. *Am. J. Clin. Nutr.* 1981; 34: 1593-1599.

[4]   de Gonzalez AB, Hartge P, Cerhan JR et al. Body-Mass Index and Mortality among 1.46 Million White Adults. *N. Engl. J. Med.* 2010; 363: 2211-2219.

[5]   Bouchard C, Shephard RJ, Stephens T. *Physical Activity, fitness and health*. Champaign, IL: Human Kinetics, 1994.

[6]   Gunther B. Dimensional analysis and the theory of biological similarity. *Physiol. Rev.* 1975; 55: 659-699.

[7]   Garn S. The applicability of North American growth standards in developing countries.*Can. Med. Assoc. J.* 1965; 93: 914-919.

[8]   Shephard RJ, Kaneko M. Ishii K. Simple indices of obesity. *J. Sports Med Phys Fitness* 1971; 11: 154-161.

[9]   Lapidus L, Bengtsson C, Larsson B et al. Distribution of adipose tissue and risk of cardiovascular disease and death: A 12-year follow-up of participants in the population study of women in Göthenburg, Sweden. *BMJ* 1984; 289: 1257-1261.

[10] Reichley KB, Mueller WH, Harris CL et al. Centralized obesity and cardiovascular disease risk in Mexican-Americans. *Am. J. Epidemiol.* 1987; 125: 373-386.

[11] Shephard RJ. *Body composition in biological anthropology*. London, UK: Cambridge University Press, 1991.

[12] Shephard RJ, Rode A. Cardio-respiratory status of the Canadian Eskimo. In: *Polar Human Biology,* eds. OG Edholm, EKE Gunderson. London, UK: Heinemann Medical Books, 1973, pp. 216-239.

[13] Nutrition Canada. Nutrition: A National Priority. Eskimo Survey Report. Ottawa, ON: Dept. of National Health and Welfare, 1975.

[14] Johnston FE, Laughlin WS, Harper AB et al. Physical growth of St. Lawrence Island Eskimos: Body size, proportions and composition. *Am. J. Phys. Anthrop.* 1982; 58: 397-401.

[15] Jamison PL. Growth of Eskimo children in Northwestern Alaska. In: *Circumpolar Health.* eds: RJ Shephard, S Itoh. Toronto, ON: University of Toronto Press, 1976; pp. 223-229.

[16] Hrdlicka A. Height and weight in Eskimo children. *Am. J. Phys. Anthropol.* 1941; 28: 331-341.

[17] Auger F, Jamison PL, Balsev-Jorgensen J et al. Anthropometry of circumpolar populations. In: *The biology of circumpolar populations,* ed: FA Milan. London, UK: Cambridge University Press, 1980; pp. 213-255.

[18] Bagust A,Walley T.An alternative to body mass index for standardizing body weight for stature. *Q J Med* 2000; 93:589-596.

[19] Norgan NG.Population differences in body composition in relation to the body mass index. *Eur. J. Clin. Nutr.* 1994;48:S10-25.

[20] Charbonneau-Roberts G, Tremblay A, Dewailly E et al. Obesity measures among Inuit of Nunavik. Arctic Net. Poster presentation at third annual meeting, Victoria, BC, 2006.

[21] Charbonneau-Roberts G, Saudny-Unterberger H, Kuhnlein HV et al. Body mass index may over-estimate the prevalence of overweight and obesity among the Inuit. *Int. J. Circumpolar Health* 2005; 64: 163-169.

[22] Becker-Christensen FG. Growth in Greenland: development of body proportions and menarcheal age in Greenlandic children. *Int. J. Circumpolar Health* 2003;62: 284-295.

[23] Young TK. Are the circumpolar inuit becoming obese? *Am. J. Hum. Biol.* 2007; 19: 181-189.

[24] Shephard RJ, Rode A. The health consequences of "modernization." *Evidence from circumpolar peoples.* London: Cambridge University Press, 1996, pp. 1-306.

[25] Godin G, Shephard RJ. Activity patterns of the Canadian Eskimo. In: *Polar Human Biology.* eds: OG Edhom, EKE Gunderson. London, UK: Heinemann Medical Books, 1973. pp. 193-215.

[26] Jørgensen ME. Obesity and metabolic correlates among the Inuit and a general Danish population. *Int..J. Circumpolar Health.* 2004;63 Suppl 2:77-79.

[27] Jørgensen ME, Glümer C, Bjerregaard P et al. Obesity and central fat pattern among Greenland Inuit and a general population of Denmark (Inter99): relationship to metabolic risk factors. *Int. J. Obes. Relat Metab. Disord.* 2003; 27:1507-1515.

[28] Jørgensen ME, Borch-Johnsen K, Bjerregaard P. Lifestyle modifies obesity-associated risk of cardiovascular disease in a genetically homogeneous population. *Am. J. Clin. Nutr.* 2006; 84:29-36.

[29] Schaefer O. Pre- and post-natal growth acceleration and increased sugar consumption in Canadian Eskimos. *Can. Med. Assoc. J.* 1970; 103: 1059-1068.

[30] Jamison P. Secular trends and the pattern of growth in arctic populations. *Soc. Sci. Med.* 1990; 30: 751-759.

[31] Heller CA, Scott EM, Hammer LM. Height, weight and growth of Alaskan Eskimos. *Am. J. Dis. Childh* 1967; 113: 338-344.

[32] Shephard RJ, Goodman J, Rode A, Schaefer O. Snowmobile use and decrease of stature among the Inuit. *Arct. Med. Res.* 1984; 38: 32-36.

[33] Petersen KM, Brant LJ. Growth and hematological changes in the Eskimo children of Wainwright, Alaska.: 1968-1977. *Am. J. Clin. Nutr.* 1984; 39: 460-465.

[34] Zammit MP. Growth patterns of Labrador Inuit youth: 1. Height and weight. *Arct .Med. Res.* 1993; 52: 153-160.

[35] Skrobak-Kaczynski J, Lewin T. Secular changes in Lapps of Northern Finland. In: *Circumpolar Health,* eds: RJ Shephard, S Itoh. Toronto: University of Toronto Press, 1976; pp: 239-247.

[36] Dangour AD, Schilg S, Hulse JA, Cole TJ. Sitting height and subischial leg length centile curves for boys and girls from Southeast England. *Ann. Hum. Biol*. 2002; 29: 290-305.

[37] Gerver WJM,De Bruin R,Drayer NM.A persisting seculartrend for body measurements in Dutch children. The Oosterwolde II study. *Acta Paediatr* 1994;83:812-814.

[38] Shephard RJ, Rode A. Growth patterns of Canadian Inuit children: a longitudinal study. *Arctic Med. Res*. 1995:60-68.

[39] Rode A, Shephard RJ. *Fitness and health of an Inuit community: 20n years of cultural change*. Ottawa, ON: Circumpolar and Scientific Affairs.

[40] Rode A, Shephard RJ. The physiological consequences of acculturation: a 20-year study in an Arctic community. *Eur. J. Appl. Physiol*. 1994; 69: 516-524.

[41] Young TK. Human obesity and arctic adaptation. Epidemiological patterns, metabolic effects and evolutionary implications. Ph.D. Dissertation, Oxford, UK: Linacre College, 1994.

[42] Young TK, Sevenhuysen G. Obesity in Northern Canadian Indians:patterns, determinants and consequences. *Am. J. Clin. Nutr*.1989; 49: 786-793.

[43] Ekoé JM, Thouez JP, Petitclerc C et al. Epidemiology of obesity in relationship to some chronic medical conditions among Inuit and Cree Indian populations in New Québec, Canada. *Diab. Res. Clin. Pract* 1990; s17-s27.

[44] Rode A, Shephard RJ, Vloshinsky PE, et al. (1995). Plasma fatty acid profiles of Canadian Inuit and Siberian nGanasan. Arct. Med. Res 1995; 54:10-20.

[45] Young TK. Sociocultural and behavioural determinants of obesity among Inuit in the central Canadian Arctic. *Soc. Sci. Med*. 1996;43:1665-1671.

[46] Young TK.Obesity,central fat patterning and their metabolic correlates among the Inuit of the Central Canadian Arctic.*Hum. Biol*. 1996;68:245-263.

[47] Young TK, Bjerregaard P, Dewailly E et al. Prevalence of Obesity and Its Metabolic Correlates Among the Circumpolar Inuit in 3 Countries. *Am. J. Public Health*. 2007; 97: 691–695.

[48] Potvin L, Desrosiers S, Trifonopolous M, et al. Anthropometric characteristics of Mohawk children aged 6 to 11 years: A population perspective. *J. Am. Diet Assoc.* 1999;99:955-61.

[49] Young TK, Dean HJ, Flett B, et al. Childhood obesity in a population at high risk for type 2 diabetes. *J. Pediatr.* 2000;136:365-369.

[50] Hanley AJ, Harris SB, Gittelsohn J et al. Overweight among children and adolescents in a Native Canadian community: Prevalence and associated factors. *Am. J. Clin. Nutr.* 2000;71:693-700.

[51] Dyck RF, Klomp H,Tan L. From "thrifty genotype" to "hefty fetal phenotype": The relationship between high birth weight and diabetes in Saskatchewan Registered Indians. *Can. J. Public Health* 2001;92:340-344.

[52] Rode A, Shephard RJ. Acculturation and the loss of fitness in the Inuit: The preventive role of active leisure. *Arct. Med. Res.* 1993; 52: 107-112.

In: New Trends in Body Mass Index Research   ISBN 978-1-61942-430-2
Editors: A. Vermeulen and E. De Smet   © 2012 Nova Science Publishers, Inc.

Chapter VI

BMI AT YOUNGER AGES AND HEALTH-RELATED QUALITY OF LIFE IN OLDER AGE

Martha L. Daviglus, Amber Pirzada and Lijing L. Yan
Department of Preventive Medicine and Medicine, Division of Geriatrics,
Northwestern University, Feinberg School of Medicine, Chicago, IL, US

ABSTRACT

Overweight/obesity (body mass index [BMI] of 25.0-29.9 and $\geq$ 30.0 kg/m^2 respectively) – now recognized as a major modifiable risk factor – is associated with higher risk of cardiovascular and non-cardiovascular morbidity and mortality, higher health care costs, and shorter life expectancy. Despite declines in prevalence of other key major cardiovascular disease (CVD) risk factors such as hypercholesterolemia, high blood pressure, and cigarette smoking, prevalence of overweight and obesity has reached epidemic proportions and continues to rise with significant implications for the future health and well being of the aging population. While the short-term effects of BMI on quality of life (i.e., physical, mental and social well-being) are well established, the impact of BMI measured earlier in life on future health-related quality of life of men and women who survive to older ages has only recently been demonstrated. This chapter presents findings on the relation of BMI measured in middle age to health-related quality of life in older age (65 years and older), after an average follow-up of 31 years, among surviving participants from the Chicago Heart Association Detection Project in Industry (CHA). The CHA study is a prospective investigation of CVD risk factors. From late 1967 to early 1973, 39,522 men and women ages 18 and older, of varied ethnicities and socioeconomic levels, employed by 84 Chicago-area organizations, were screened. In 1996 and 2001, quality of life was assessed with widely used and standardized instruments, i.e., 12-item Health Status Questionnaire (HSQ-12), Medical Outcomes Trust 36-item Short-Form Health Survey (SF-36) performance of activities of daily living (ADL), and instrumental activities of daily living (IADL). Results demonstrate that higher BMI in middle age adversely impacts future health-related quality of life and physical functioning in older age. Conversely, for non-overweight persons (BMI 18.5-24.9 kg/m^2), preservation of health status and quality of life is evident, indicating that increasing life expectancy can be accompanied with disease-free and disability-free survival. With adverse BMI levels afflicting a large proportion of the US population and increasing numbers of people surviving to older ages, preventive measures are urgently required at younger ages to lessen future individual and societal burden of disease, health care costs, and also disability and impaired quality of life associated with excess weight.

INTRODUCTION

Overweight/ obesity (body mass index [BMI] of 25.0 – 29.9 and ≥ 30.0 kg/m^2 respectively) – recently recognized in a statement by the American Heart Association [Eckel RH et al., 1998] as a major modifiable cardiovascular disease risk factor – is associated with higher risk of coronary heart disease (CHD) and cardiovascular disease (CVD) morbidity and mortality and all-cause mortality, and shorter life expectancy among middle-aged and older individuals, as well as with increased risk of morbidity from hypertension, diabetes, dyslipidemia, musculoskeletal problems, and other disorders [NHLBI Obesity Initiative Expert Panel, 1998]. Recent reports based on large cohorts of young adult men and women with decades of follow-up have demonstrated that BMI measured even in young adulthood is related to higher risk of mortality from cardiovascular diseases and all causes [Dyer AR et al., 2004; Priyanath A et al., 2001]. Furthermore, higher BMI has been associated with higher health care costs, both cross-sectionally and in prospective investigations, and it has been estimated that obesity-related morbidity accounts for 5.7% of total health care expenditures in the United States [Wolf AM and Colditz GA, 1998].

Despite declines in prevalence of other key major CVD risk factors – hypercholesterolemia, high blood pressure, and cigarette smoking – in the last few decades [Cooper R et al., 2000], the prevalence of overweight and obesity has increased markedly over the same period in all age groups in the US and other countries and it continues to rise with profound implications for the future health and well being of the aging population. From the early 1970s to early 1990's, obesity prevalence increased from 10.2% to 14.9% among men, and from 12.3% to 20.6% among women; findings from recent surveys and data from the 1999-2000 National Health and Nutrition Examination Survey (NHANES) show that adverse BMI trends have persisted with further increases in age-specific and age-adjusted prevalence of overweight and obesity [Kuczmarski RJ et al., 1994; Flegal KM et al., 1998; Flegal KM et al., 2002]. Currently, approximately 130 million American adults are overweight or obese [American Heart Association 2003]. Disturbingly, similar trends have been observed in children and adolescents [Troiano RP and Flegal KM, 1998; Ogden CL et al., 2002], and deleterious consequences of obesity such as non-insulin dependent diabetes mellitus are becoming increasingly common in these and other age groups [Rosenbloom AL et al., 1999; Sinha R et al., 2002].

BMI AND HEALTH-RELATED QUALITY OF LIFE AND DISABILITY

While the consequences of obesity have been extensively examined among young and middle-aged individuals and among study populations comprised of a wide range of age groups, less attention has focused on the impact of obesity among older people. Moreover, although research interest has focused on predictors of health-related quality of life in older age in recent years, most data on the relationship between BMI and quality of life are from cross-sectional studies. The few existing long-term studies have focused mainly on physical functioning and there are still some uncertainties regarding the association between excess weight and quality of life. The aging of the US population and the functional impairment and declining quality of life that often accompany advancing age necessitate further examination of this important and modifiable risk factor.

Cross-Sectional Studies on Relationship of BMI and Quality of Life

Cross-sectional studies on effect of BMI on quality of life conducted to date have generally demonstrated a negative impact of overweight and obesity on some aspects of quality of life [Chambers BA et al., 2002; Coakley EH et al., 1998; Doll HA et al., 2000; Ford ES et al., 2001; Galanos AN et al., 1994; Han TS et al., 1998; Katz DA et al., 2000; Lean MEJ et al., 1999; Lopez-Garcia E et al., 2003; Sternfeld B et al., 2002; Yan LL et al., 2004; Yancy WS et al., 2002]. However, these studies have mostly included mixed age groups. In a cross-sectional study of 1,885 men and 2,156 women ages 20 – 59 years from the Netherlands, high BMI was associated with increased risk of impairment in quality of life and physical functioning. With adjustment for age, and demographic and lifestyle factors, individuals with BMI in the highest tertile were about twice as likely to have poor physical functioning (score < 66.7%) compared to those in the lowest BMI tertile and were also more likely to report bodily pain and poor general health (women only). Compared to those in the lowest BMI tertile, men and women in the highest tertile were significantly more likely to have difficulties in performing a range of basic daily activities such as climbing several flight of stairs [Odd Ratios (ORs) and 95% Confidence Intervals (CI) for men and women were 2.03, 1.43 – 2.88 and 2.09, 1.58 – 2.77], or walking more than 1 km (men: 1.93, 1.35 – 2.74; women: 1.77, 1.32 – 2.39). Women with adverse BMI levels generally had more severe difficulties than men in performing basic activities of daily living. Similar results were obtained with measures of waist circumference and waist-to-hip ratios. However, findings for social and mental health-related quality of life did not differ significantly by weight category. Quality of life was assessed using the Dutch version of the RAND-36 questionnaire – an adaptation of the standardized 36-item Short-Form (SF-36) Health Survey – which captures nine health concepts including measures of functioning, i.e., ability to perform daily tasks and activities and measures of well-being, i.e., subjective assessment of physical and emotional health and general health perceptions [Han TS et al., 1998]. Similar associations with physical functioning were obtained when the BMI classification adopted by the National Institutes of Health was used [Lean MEJ et al., 1999].

A cross-sectional postal survey of 8,889 randomly selected British men and women ages 18 – 64 years in 1997 included questions on weight and height, chronic diseases, and the SF-36 questionnaire developed by the Medical Outcomes Study (MOS) that provides eight dimensions or domains of physical, emotional, and social well-being. Normal weight individuals (BMI 18.5 – 24.9 kg/m^2) had significantly higher scores in each physical well-being dimension compared to overweight participants. Persons with moderate to morbid obesity (BMI 30.0 – 39.9 and $\geq$ 40.0 kg/m^2, respectively) had significantly lower scores in dimensions of physical well-being (Physical Functioning, Role-Physical, Bodily Pain) than those in all other BMI categories including those who were underweight. Scores of morbidly obese participants were lower than those who were moderately obese although the difference was significant only for Physical Functioning (mean difference in score 14.2 $\pm$ 2.4; 95% CI, 7.6 – 20.9). In the emotional and social well-being dimensions, normal weight and overweight participants had the highest scores with scores of overweight slightly higher in all dimensions except Vitality. Mean scores of moderately and morbidly obese individuals were generally similar to those of underweight individuals. In the presence of chronic illnesses, obesity was associated with additional significant deterioration in physical but not in emotional well-being [Doll HA et al., 2000]. In a cross-sectional analysis of data on 2,931 MOS participants mean age 54.9 $\pm$ 15 years, with chronic medical and psychiatric conditions, quality of life was assessed using the SF-36 questionnaire. Overweight persons (BMI 25.0 – 29.9 kg/m^2) and those with class I or class II/ III obesity (BMI of 30.0 – 34.9 and $\geq$ 35 kg/m^2 respectively) had significantly lower scores for Physical Functioning (by 3.4, 7.8, and 13.8 points, respectively), Role Limitations due to Physical Health, and Bodily Pain, and obese persons had significantly lower Health Perception (by 2.8, and 4.4 points for obesity class I and II/III), and Vitality measures (by 4.0 and 7.1 points) compared to normal weight individuals with adjustment for demographic factors, health habits, medical conditions, and depression. Women with higher BMI had significantly lower quality of life in several domains compared to men, as did blacks with higher BMI (especially for mental health measures) compared to whites [Katz DA et al., 2000].

Coakley et al. reported that among 56,510 women ages 45 – 71 years from the Nurses' Health Study, there was a significant, graded inverse association between BMI and physical functioning assessed using the MOS SF-36 questionnaire. On average, women with BMI levels of 30 – 34.9 kg/m^2 had lower scores for Physical Functioning, Vitality, and Bodily Pain by 9.0 points (95% CI -9.5 – -8.5), 5.6 points (95% CI, -6.1 – -5.1), and 7.0 points (95% CI, -7.6 – -6.4), i.e., approximately 10% lower functioning compared to women with BMI from 22.0 – 23.9 kg/m^2. Heavier women were at 66% higher risk of limitations in ability to work or perform other roles (relative risk = 1.66; 95% CI, 1.56 - 1.76). In stepwise regression analyses including age, physical activity,smoking status, alcohol consumption, and chronic illness variables, BMI was the most important predictor of physical functioning and bodily pain, and the second most important predictor of vitality after physical activity. Similar findings were obtained when analyses were limited to women who had maintained their BMI over a ten-year period. [Coakley EH et al., 1998]. Among 1,168 male outpatients ages 45 – 65 years (mean age 54.7 ± 5.6) attending the Durham Veterans' Affairs Medical Center, those with BMI > 40 kg/m^2 had significantly lower (by ≥ 5 points) SF-36 domain scores compared with normal weight individuals, for Physical Functioning, Role-Physical, Bodily Pain, and Vitality and for the Physical Component Summary score, with adjustment for age, race, comorbidities, depression, and physical activity. BMI of 35 to 40 kg/m^2 was also associated with significantly lower scores for Physical Functioning and Bodily Pain domains and Physical Component Summary scores, compared to normal weight men [Yancy WS et al., 2002].

The 1996 Behavioral Risk Factor Surveillance System Survey (BRFSS) also included a set of four health-related quality of life questions developed by the Centers for Disease Control (CDC) as a brief and validated measure for surveillance of physical and mental health trends and disparities in general populations. These include assessment of general health perception, number of unhealthy days in the last month with regards to physical health and to mental health, and number of days in the last month with limitations in usual activity due to poor health, either physical or mental. Among the 109,076 respondents (47,066 men and 62,010 women ages 18 years and older) who had complete data on BMI, quality of life measures, and other key variables, BMI had a U-shaped relation with all measures of quality of life, with the 18.5 to < 25 kg/m^2 group generally having the lowest (best) mean values for the above quality of life measures. General health perception, physical health, mental health, and limitation of activities worsened when BMI increased above this range or decreased below it. For example, compared with persons with BMI of 18.5 to < 25 kg/m^2, likelihood of having poor or fair self-rated health was higher among underweight persons (OR 1.57, 95% CI, 1.31 – 1.89) and also increased with increasing BMI (ORs and 95% CIs were 1.12 [1.04 – 1.20], 1.65 [1.50 – 1.81], 2.58 [2.21 – 3.00], and 3.23 [2.63 – 3.95], respectively for BMI groups 25 to < 30, 30 to < 35, 35 to < 40, and ≥ 40 kg/m^2). These relationships were only slightly affected by adjustment for age, gender, race or ethnicity, education, employment, smoking status, and physical activity [Ford ES et al., 2001].

Another much smaller cross-sectional study (51 men and 80 women from southwestern Ohio) of a broad age range (20 to 86 years) showed that having high levels of all major CVD risk factors, including obesity, was associated with lower quality of life assessed using the MOS SF-36 questionnaire. β-coefficients for the relation of obesity (BMI $\geq$ 30 kg/m^2) to SF-36 scores were negative (indicating the adverse effect of obesity) for three of eight dimensions of quality of life, i.e., Physical Functioning, General Health, and Vitality, with associations significant for Physical Functioning and General Health ($p <$ 0.05) [Chambers BA et al., 2002]. In a study relating body composition to functional impairment, Sternfeld et al. examined cross-sectional associations of measures of fat and lean mass with physical performance – assessed by walking speed and grip strength – and self-reported functional limitation (assessed by 10 questions on the degree of difficulty in various physical functions such as stooping, lifting or carrying more than 10 pounds, and walking up and down stairs). Among 708 men and 947 women ages 55 and older from Sonoma, California, higher fat mass was associated with slower walking speed and higher chance of self-reported functional limitations, suggesting that fat mass adversely impacts some aspects of physical performance and functioning [Sternfeld B et al., 2002]. Among 81,787 adult BRFSS respondents ages 45 years and older, those with BMI $\geq$ 40 kg/m^2 (class III obesity) both with and without self-reported arthritis, were significantly more likely to report disability (assessed by two questions asking whether the participant is limited in any activities because of physical, mental, or emotional problems, and whether the participant has any health problem that requires the use of special equipment). Compared with normal weight persons, odds ratios and 95% confidence intervals for disability for those with class III obesity were 2.75 (2.22 – 3.40) and 1.77 (1.20 – 2.62) among those with and without self-reported arthritis. Among those with arthritis, overweight women and men and women with class I and class II obesity also had higher odds of disability [Okoro CA et al., 2004].

There is limited research on the relationship of BMI and quality of life among older adults. In the Chicago Heart Association Detection Project in Industry (CHA) study, surviving participants ages 65 and older were mailed a follow-up health survey in 1996, which included assessment of health-related quality of life using the 12-item Health Status Questionnaire (HSQ-12) [Health Outcomes Institute, 1996]. BMI in 1996 was computed from self-reported weight and height. Among the 3,981 men and 3,099 women who responded and had complete data on quality of life and other key variables, obesity (BMI $\geq$ 30.0 kg/m^2) was associated with lower health perception and poorer physical and social functioning (women only). No significant differences in mental health domains were found between obese persons and others. Overweight (BMI 25.0 – 29.9 kg/m^2) was associated with impaired physical well-being among women only. Underweight men and women reported impairment in physical, social and mental well-being. Associations were independent of age, race, education, smoking, and alcohol intake, and were attenuated but not eliminated with further adjustment for comorbidities [Yan LL et al., 2004]. In a small clinical study of 88 older women (mean age 71 ± 4.9 years) participating in a nutrition screening program in Pennsylvania, physical function was assessed by performance of 18 physical tasks which included writing a sentence, lifting a book, picking a penny from the floor, climbing stairs, and walking 50 feet. Higher BMI was significantly associated with poorer performance of these physical tasks assessing upper and lower body function. For example, median time to walk 50 feet was 17.0, 17.6, and 19.1 seconds for women with BMI of 22 to < 27, 27 to < 30, and ≥ 30 kg/m^2 respectively [Apovian CM et al., 2002].

Another report examined the relation of sub-optimal health-related quality of life (defined as a score less than 100) on each SF-36 domain with BMI, among 3,605 non-institutionalized Spanish men and women ages 60 and older. Compared to normal weight participants, prevalence of sub-optimal physical functioning was higher among obese persons (BMI ≥ 30.0 kg/m^2) with adjustment for sociodemographic variables, tobacco and alcohol consumption, physical activity, hypertension and diagnosis of chronic diseases (for men: OR, 1.91; 95% CI, 1.22 – 3.00; for women: OR, 2.58; 95% CI, 1.59 – 4.19). Aspects of physical functioning that were most affected were bending, kneeling or stooping, climbing stairs and strenuous effort. Of note, obesity was associated with better mental health-related quality of life for men but not for women. Similar results were obtained for both participants ages 60 – 74 years and those ages 75 and older [Lopez Garcia E et al., 2003]. In the NHANES I Epidemiologic Follow-Up Study (NHEFS; 1982-84), functional impairment was assessed by a 26-item battery compiled from the Fries Functional Disability Scale for Arthritis, the Rosow-Breslau Scale, and the Katz Activities of Daily Living Scale. Among 3,053 community-dwelling men and women ages 65 – 85 years, those with high or low BMI were at greater risk of functional impairment. Compared to those with BMI in the 15th – 85th percentile for the cohort, individuals with BMI ≤ 15th percentile or ≥ 85th percentile were 34% and 43% more likely to have functional impairment (ORs and 95% CIs were 1.34 [1.04 – 1.74] and 1.43 [1.10 – 1.86] respectively) with adjustment for age, sex, self-rated health, presence of chronic diseases, and other potential confounders [Galanos AN et al., 1994].

The cross-sectional design of these studies and the broad age range of samples preclude any inference as to the causal effect of BMI on health-related quality of life in older population strata. A possible explanation for the observed lack of associations of BMI with emotional health or social well-being in these studies may be the inclusion of younger persons, for whom sufficient time had not elapsed for adverse effects of high BMI levels to become apparent.

Long-Term Relationship of BMI and Quality of Life

The few longitudinal studies on quality of life [Daviglus ML et al., 2003; Ferraro KF et al., 2002; Harris TB et al., 1997; Jenkins KR et al., 2004; Launer LJ et al., 1994; Visscher TL et al., 2004] have mainly focused on the effect of BMI on physical disability and performance of activities of daily living and not on the entire spectrum of quality of life involving physical, mental, and social aspects of life [Tibblin G, 1993]. Ferraro, et al. utilized data from NHANES I (1971-75) and the NHEFS (conducted in 2 waves of follow-up in 1982-84 and 1992) to assess relation between baseline BMI and disability after 10 and 20 years (using upper-body and lower-body disability indices comprised of physical tasks such as dressing/ grooming, and eating to assess upper body disability; hygiene and toileting and walking to assess lower body disability), among 6,833 persons ages 25 – 74 years at baseline. They reported higher long-term risk of upper- and especially lower-body disability for persons who were obese at baseline, but no consistent relationship of overweight to higher disability. Persons who were normal weight at baseline but became obese also had higher disability at both 10 and 20 years of follow-up. Of note, persons who were obese at baseline but subsequently become normal weight did not experience a reduction in their disability, indicating that obesity has a lasting effect on disability [Ferraro KF et al., 2002].

Similarly, another study using data from NHANES I on 1,124 white women ages 45 years and older at baseline (1971-75) found that having a BMI in the highest tertile either at baseline or in 1982-84 (current BMI) was associated with higher incident mobility disability through 1987. Mobility disability was defined as self-reported disability in performance of at least one of several activities, walking a quarter of a mile, walking across a room, climbing two steps, doing heavy chores, carrying a full bag of groceries, running errands, bending to the floor or transferring from a car, bed, bath, chair or toilet. For both young-old (n = 698; baseline ages 45 – 59 years) and old-old women (n = 426; baseline ages 60 – 74 years) those with high baseline BMI (i.e., > 27.0 and > 28.1 respectively) were at twice the risk of disability compared to women with low baseline BMI (ORs and 95% CIs for young-old and old-old women with high baseline BMI were 2.38 [1.44 – 3.93] and 2.04 [1.20 – 3.49]). Among young-old women only, current BMI (i.e., measured 2 to 5 years prior to disability ascertainment) was as strongly related to disability as baseline BMI [Launer LJ et al., 1994]. In the Cardiovascular Health Study (CHS) of 4,800 older American men and women, both higher self-reported weight at age 50 (15 years or more before initial examination) and higher current weight at age 65+ years (i.e., weight in the fourth quartile for the cohort) were associated with poorer health status especially among women. Heavier persons had poorer self-reported health (based on a question on global health status), more mobility difficulty (both self-reported and with measured walking time), and were taking more medications [Harris TB et al., 1997]. Using data from 2 waves of the Asset and Health Dynamics Among the Oldest Old (AHEAD) survey, 1995 and 1998, Jenkins KR showed that among men and women ages 70 years and older at baseline, those who were obese in 1993 were significantly more likely to experience onset of impairment in strength and lower body mobility (but not upper body mobility) over the next 3 years. Compared to normal weight individuals, with adjustment for socio-demographic factors and various health behaviors and conditions, odds of onset of strength impairment among overweight and obese individuals were 1.48 (95% CI: 1.15 – 1.91) and 2.17 (95% CI: 1.32 – 3.56) respectively, and odds of onset of impairment in lower body mobility were 1.48 (95% CI: 1.08 – 2.03) and 2.07 (95% CI: 1.31 – 3.27), respectively [Jenkins KR, 2004].

Among 19,518 Finnish men and women ages 20 – 92 years who were followed for 15 years, obesity at baseline (i.e., BMI $\geq$ 30 kg/m^2) was associated with a higher number of unhealthy life-years assessed by work disability (i.e., receiving any work disability pension and assessed for participants ages 20 – 64 years at baseline), CHD, and long-term medication use. Compared to their normal weight counterparts, obese men ages 20 – 64 years who never smoked had on average, 0.63 more years of work disability, 0.36 more years of CHD, and 1.68 more years of long-term medication use; corresponding figures for women were 0.52, 0.46, and 1.49 more unhealthy life-years. Obese men and women generally had higher risks of work disability, CHD, and need for long-term medication (for example, compared to normal-weight men and women, relative risks for work disability for obese men and women ages 20 – 64 were 2.3 [95% CI, 1.6 – 3.4] and 1.6 [95% CI, 1.4 – 2.0]). Excess risks of obesity-related disease and disability were highest in the youngest age groups, highlighting the lasting impact of early-onset obesity [Visscher TL et al., 2004].

In the CHA study (see below for more details of the study), a health survey was mailed in 1996 after an average 26 years of follow-up to all surviving participants ages 65 years and older with current addresses (n = 12,409) obtained from the Health Care Financing Administration (HCFA, now the Centers for Medicare and Medicaid Services [CMS]). The questionnaire included self-reports of risk factors, health-related quality of life assessed using the HSQ-12 questionnaire, habitual exercise pattern, alcohol consumption, smoking history, history of diseases and conditions, and current medication use for hypertension, hypercholesterolemia, diabetes, and hormone replacement therapy (for women). The response rate was 59.8%; average follow-up was 25.8 years for all respondents.

For the 6,766 men and women ages 36 - 64 years without diabetes mellitus or myocardial infarction at baseline, who completed the 26 year follow-up questionnaire at ages 65 or older, baseline BMI had significant, inverse, graded associations with all aspects of quality of life (physical, social and mental well-being) in older age. Among normal weight individuals, preservation of health status was evident in the physical, emotional and social domains. There was an inverse graded association between BMI and all eight HSQ-12 domains scores for men and women, i.e., scores were highest (best) in individuals with BMI of 18.5 to < 25.0 kg/m^2 and decreased significantly with higher BMI, with worst outcomes for obese persons (BMI $\geq$ 30.0 kg/m^2) after adjustment for baseline CVD risk factors and age in 1996. For example, normal weight women had an adjusted Health Perception score of 63.7, which was 7.0 and 15.5 points higher than overweight and obese women respectively. In general, the inverse associations were stronger for physical health than for mental health or social well-being. Tests for linear trend showed that all trends were statistically significant (p-values ranged from 0.006 to < 0.001). A higher multivariate-adjusted percentage of normal weight persons also reported no limitation in common basic physical activities, and perceived themselves as having excellent or very good health compared with overweight and obese persons (for women, 46.8% vs. 37.9% and 24.3%; for men, 53.8% vs. 49.1% and 36.5%; p-values for trend < 0.001). These findings demonstrate that high BMI levels do have significant long-term adverse effects, not only on physical health, but also on emotional and social health, although to a lesser degree [Daviglus ML et al., 2003]. Results from the CHA cohort regarding health perception are remarkably similar to the CHS, i.e., excess weight in middle age was related to poorer health status in older age. As in the CHS, results from the CHA follow-up survey show that compared to normal weight participants, higher percentages of overweight and obese participants (44.6%, vs. 55.1%, and 69.1%, respectively) were taking medications for blood pressure, cholesterol, or diabetes, which may also have influenced quality of life. Thus, overweight and obesity in middle age appear to impair numerous aspects of quality of life in older age. Ferraro et al. examined both cross-sectional and longitudinal associations between BMI and measures of functional illness using data from Americans' Changing Lives, a longitudinal study of 3,617 non-institutionalized men and women ages 25 and older at baseline in 1986. Obesity was cross-sectionally associated with higher levels of functional impairment (assessed using the four-category Guttman scale of self-reported impairment ranging from 1, i.e., no major impairment, to 4, i.e., currently in bed or chair and/or high difficulty bathing), and functional limitation (i.e., extent to which daily activities are limited by health or health-related problems). In longitudinal analyses (limited to three years of follow-up), obesity was not associated with change in functional impairment, but obese respondents did experience a significant increase in functional limitation over time [Ferraro KF and Booth TL, 1999].

While Yan LL et al. found no cross-sectional association between obesity and mental health at ages 65 years and older among CHA participants, longitudinal data from the CHA cohort on BMI measured in midlife and quality of life in older age revealed a dose-response increase in impairment of social functioning and mental health domains, although less strongly than impairment of physical health domains [Yan LL et al., 2004; Daviglus ML et al., 2003].

One possible explanation for the different cross-sectional and longitudinal findings is that some individuals may have gained weight in the few years prior to assessment of quality of life, and were classified in the obese group in the report by Yan et al. Thus, duration of exposure may have been too short for the adverse effects of obesity to become apparent, especially in the social and mental health domains. Among CHA participants, 43% of men and 47% of women who were obese at follow-up reported a weight gain of more than 10 pounds in the last 10 years, compared to 18% and 8% of normal weight men and women, respectively [Yan LL et al., 2004].

Hence, while the short-term effects of BMI on quality of life (i.e., physical, mental and social well-being) are well established, the impact of BMI measured in middle age on future health-related quality of life of men and women who survive to older ages (65 years and older) has only recently been demonstrated, based on long-term follow-up of the CHA Study, with quality of life assessed using a 12-item questionnaire.

Here we present new population-based findings on the relation of BMI measured in middle-aged employed men and women to subsequent physical, mental and social health-related quality of life and self-reported disability assessed in older age using the widely used and well validated SF-36 questionnaire, activities of daily living and instrumental activities of daily living, and with follow-up extended to an average of 31 years, among surviving participants from the CHA Study.

THE CHICAGO HEART ASSOCIATION DETECTION PROJECT IN INDUSTRY

Participants and Baseline Examination

The CHA study is a prospective investigation of the impact of CVD risk factors. Between November 1967 and January 1973, the CHA study screened 39,522 women and men ages 18 years and older of varied ethnicities and socioeconomic levels.

All employees of 84 Chicago-area companies and organizations, about 75,000 people, were invited to participate; volunteer rate was 53%. Details of the baseline examination have been reported [Stamler J et al., 1975; Stamler J et al., 1993]. Screening was performed by two trained and standardized four-person field teams. Height and weight were measured with calibrated research equipment with participants in light indoor clothing.

A single casual supine blood pressure was obtained using a standard mercury sphygmomanometer, and a non-fasting blood sample was analyzed by an automated adaptation of the method of Levine and Zak for determination of serum total cholesterol [Levine JB and Zak B, 1964]. All measurements were collected in a standardized way, using a single protocol with uniform methods at all screening sites.

A self-administered questionnaire was used to collect demographic data, smoking history, and information on medical diagnoses and treatment of hypercholesterolemia, hypertension, diabetes, and myocardial infarction (MI). Resting electrocardiograms (ECGs) were taken and results classified as having major, minor only, or no abnormalities based on criteria of the national cooperative Pooling Project and the Hypertension Detection and Follow-up Program [The Pooling Project Research Group, 1978; Prineas RJ et al., 1983]. Vital status was ascertained through 2000, with average follow-up of 30 years. Deaths were determined by several methods: before 1979, by direct mail, telephone, contact with employer, matching of cohort records with Social Security Administration files; and after 1979, by matching of study records with National Death Index (NDI) records.

31-Year Follow-Up Questionnaires

A second follow-up questionnaire was mailed in 2001, to all known surviving CHA participants ages 65 and older for whom current addresses were available (n = 13,605). Current addresses were obtained from CMS by matching records with name, sex, date of birth, and social security number. As mandated by CMS, an introductory letter was first mailed to all participants informing them about the forthcoming questionnaire and emphasizing the voluntary nature of the study. Institutional review board approval to contact participants by mail 31 years after the baseline examination was received. The eight-page questionnaire included self-reports of risk factors, health-related quality of life assessed with the widely used, MOS SF-36 questionnaire, performance of activities of daily living (ADL), and instrumental activities of daily living (IADL), habitual exercise pattern, alcohol consumption, smoking history (never, former, or currently smoking 1 to 9, 10 to 19, or 20 or more cigarettes per day), history of diseases and conditions from a checklist of 30 physician-diagnosed medical conditions (e.g., cancer by site, myocardial infarction, angina, congestive heart failure, stroke, diabetes), current medication use for hypertension, hypercholesterolemia, diabetes, and hormone replacement therapy (for women). Of the 13,605 participants who were mailed a questionnaire, 134 were reported deceased by their next-of-kin. The response rate was 58.7% with an average follow-up of about 31 years for all respondents.

Exclusions

Of the 7,910 participants (3,277 women and 4,633 men) ages 65 years and older in 2001 who completed the questionnaire, 937 were excluded for the following reasons: baseline age $\geq$ 65 years (n = 13), history of MI (n = 41) or diagnosis of diabetes (n = 158) at baseline, missing data on baseline height or weight (n = 4), missing data on blood pressure, serum cholesterol, smoking status, or education (n = 46), missing SF-36 measures at follow-up (n = 675). Additionally, 65 participants (56 women and 9 men) who were underweight at baseline, i.e., BMI < 18.5 kg/m^2, were excluded from the cohort due to small numbers in this category. Thus, the following findings are based on 4,133 men and 2,775 women ages 65 years and older in 2001 with complete data on baseline risk factors and follow-up measures of quality of life.

Baseline BMI Classification

Using BMI categories adopted by the National Institutes of Health [NHLBI Obesity Initiative Expert Panel, 1998], participants were grouped according to baseline BMI levels as normal weight (BMI 18.5 to < 25 kg/m^2), overweight (BMI 25 to < 30 kg/m^2), and obese (BMI $\geq$30 kg/m^2). Primary analyses were based on these three BMI categories. Obese participants were further subdivided into two groups: obesity class I (BMI 30 to < 35 kg/m^2) and obesity classes II/ III (severely obese, BMI $\geq$ 35 kg/m^2), and additional analyses were conducted using four BMI groups (including normal and overweight categories).

Follow-Up Measures of Quality of Life and Disability

Self-reported SF-36 questionnaire was used to measure quality of life. Validity and reliability of the SF-36 in measuring quality of life in older individuals have been demonstrated [Ware JE et al., 1995, Walters SJ et al., 2001]. The SF-36, a brief questionnaire whose 36 items are combined together to form eight dimensions, was designed to provide measures of physical functioning, i.e., ability to perform daily tasks and activities; mental health, i.e., subjective evaluation of one's own physical and emotional well-being; and social functioning, i.e., degree to which physical or emotional problems interfere with individual social activities. The SF-36 captures eight domains of health: 1) Physical Functioning (10 items), 2) Role Limitations due to Physical Health (4 items), 3) Social Functioning (2 items), 4) Bodily Pain (2 items), 5) General Mental Health (5 items), 6) Role Limitations due to Emotional Problems (3 items), 7) Vitality (4 items), and 8) General Health Perceptions (5 items). For each domain, categorical responses are coded, summed, and transformed into numeric scores ranging from 0 to 100 according to the SF-36 scoring protocol [Ware JE Jr. et al., 1993; Ware JE et al., 1995], with higher scores indicating better outcomes. Two summary health measures – a Physical Component Summary (PCS) and a Mental Component Summary (MCS) – that aggregate conceptually related health measures, were further calculated from the item scores. The total score was computed as the sum of the PCS and MCS scores.

In addition, disability was assessed using self-reports of ADL and IADLs. First defined by Katz [Katz S et al., 1963], ADL and IADL are used to determine self-care capacity. The ADL encompass six basic functions – bathing, dressing, toileting, transfer (i.e., getting in and out of bed), continence, and feeding – and provide an objective method of classifying individuals with chronic illnesses, disabilities and impairments [Katz S, 1976]. The IADL expand assessment to homemaking skills necessary for independent living [Duke University Center for the Study of Aging and Human Development, 1978; Rosow I and Breslau N, 1966], and include preparation of a simple meal; use of the telephone; shopping; money management; heavy housework such as vacuuming and mopping; and light housework such as dusting and straightening up.

Statistical Analyses

All analyses by baseline BMI groups were done separately for women and men. Chi-square (for categorical variables) or F-tests (for continuous variables) were used to detect statistically significant differences in baseline characteristics across the groups. General linear models (GLM) were used to compute group mean domain scores and summary scores adjusted for age (in 2001), race (African American or not), and the following variables assessed at baseline: education (years), cigarette smoking (number/ day), and minor and major ECG abnormalities (yes/ no). The BMI groups were entered in the linear models as a class variable. Adjusting for the same set of variables, we also computed the prevalence (%) of favorable ("good") outcomes and adverse ("bad") outcomes for representative SF-36 items from the eight domains by

BMI category using GLM. These values are covariate-adjusted least squares estimates. In addition to age, race, baseline education, cigarette smoking, and ECG abnormalities, SF-36 mean domain scores were adjusted for baseline systolic blood pressure and serum cholesterol, which are major CVD risk factors potentially in the causal pathway between BMI and health outcomes. To test for linear trend, we included BMI as a continuous variable in multivariate models (with the same set of variables) using linear regression for continuous outcomes (for example, domain scores) and logistic regression for binary outcomes (for example, prevalence of favorable outcomes). Age-adjusted prevalence (%) of having any chronic disability – ADL disability or institutionalization, and IADL disability only – was calculated by baseline BMI category, and Chi-square tests were used to detect statistically significant differences in prevalence of disability across BMI groups. All analyses were conducted using SAS statistical software (v8.02, SAS Institute Inc., Cary, NC).

FINDINGS OF THE 31-YEAR FOLLOW-UP SURVEY

Characteristics of Study Participants at Baseline

Table 1 presents baseline characteristics of study participants by BMI group for men and women separately. Women with normal weight compared to those overweight and obese were on average slightly younger, had lower average systolic and diastolic blood pressure, and lower average serum cholesterol at baseline. Other baseline characteristics were also putatively more favorable for normal weight women; for example, they had higher education levels and lower prevalence of minor ECG abnormalities. However, proportion of smokers was higher among women with normal weight: 32% were smokers, smoking on average 18 cigarettes per day, compared to 23% of overweight and 22% of obese women. Similar results for baseline characteristics were observed among men (Table 1). However, while a higher proportion of normal weight men also smoked (i.e., 33% compared to 30% of overweight men and 27% of obese men), the number of cigarettes smoked per day was higher, but not significantly, among obese male smokers (average of about 24 cigarettes per day) compared to normal weight male smokers (average 22 cigarettes per day).

SF-36 Scores

Unadjusted means, standard deviations, medians, and inter-quartile ranges of SF-36 domain scores and summary scores for men and women separately are shown in Table 2. Mean PCS and MCS scores for CHA participants were in general, slightly higher than U.S. norms, i.e., 45.5 ± 10.6 and 55.1 ± 7.6 for CHA male participants compared to 42.0 ± 11.4 and 52.5 ± 9.8 for men ages 65 years and older from the general U.S. population; 41.1 ± 12.1 and 53.9 ± 9.4 for CHA female participants compared to 41.0 ± 11.5 and 51.4 ± 10.5 for women ages 65 years and older from the general U.S. population [Ware JE Jr. et al., 1993].

Multivariate-adjusted mean scores for the eight SF-36 domains, mean PCS and MCS scores, and the total score by BMI group and gender are shown in Table 3. There was a significant inverse graded association between BMI and seven of eight SF-36 domain scores for both men and women, with adjustment for age (2001), race, education, numbers of cigarettes smoked per day, and presence of any ECG abnormalities.

For example, women with normal weight had an adjusted General Health score of 69.1, which is, respectively, 4.1 and 12.0 points higher than overweight or obese women. In general, the inverse associations were stronger for physical health (i.e., Physical Functioning, Physical Role Limitations, Bodily Pain) than for mental or social well-being. Tests for linear trend showed that all trends except those for the Mental Health domain were statistically significant at $p < 0.001$ for both men and women. While there was an inverse graded association of BMI with Mental Health domain scores among women, these findings were not significant. Among men, there was no graded association between BMI and Mental Health scores, although scores for obese men were significantly lower by 1.7 points than those for normal weight men (p-value < 0.05).

Similar results were seen for the summary scores: there was a significant, graded inverse association of BMI with the PCS score and also the total score (p-values for trends were < 0.001) but not with the MCS score for both men and women. Additional adjustment for obesity-related major CVD risk factors, serum cholesterol and blood pressure had little effect on mean SF-36 domain scores (data not shown); tests for linear trend remained significant for both genders.

We also computed the prevalence (%) of favorable ("good") outcomes and adverse ("bad") outcomes for representative SF-36 items from the eight domains by BMI category, with adjustment for age (at follow-up), race, and baseline education, cigarette smoking, and presence of ECG abnormalities.

For individual quality of life items related to physical and social health, prevalence of good outcomes was generally highest for normal weight groups and decreased with higher BMI. On the other hand, prevalence of bad outcomes was generally lower for men and women with BMI < 25 kg/m^2 and increased with higher BMI.

For example, a higher proportion of men and women with BMI < 25 kg/m^2 reported excellent or very good health compared to those overweight and obese (for women, 44.4% vs. 36.7% and 24.7% respectively; for men, 56.0% vs. 49.6% and 37.8% respectively; p-values for comparisons with normal weight group < 0.001).

Conversely, proportions of men and women who reported fair or poor health were lower among normal weight individuals compared to those overweight, and obese (for women 16.8% vs. 23.9% and 35.1% respectively; for men 12.5% vs. 14.6% and 21.8% respectively; p-values < 0.001). Similar results were seen with items dealing with Physical Functioning, i.e., performance of physical activities: lifting or carrying groceries, climbing stairs, and walking several blocks, with a consistently higher prevalence of good outcomes and lower prevalence of bad outcomes associated with lower BMI. For example, 82.1% of normal weight men reported no limitations due to health in carrying groceries compared to 77.7% of overweight and 66.2% of obese men; corresponding figures for women were 59.0%, 49.8%, and 35.5%, respectively. Conversely, only 4.9% of normal weight men reported a lot of limitations in carrying groceries compared to 6.1% of overweight and 9.7% of obese men; corresponding figures for women were 12.6%, 15.6%, and 28.6%, respectively (most p-values < 0.001). No such relationships were observed for items related to mental health.

Additional analyses using four baseline BMI strata, i.e., normal weight, overweight, obese, and severely obese, also showed a graded and inverse relationship between BMI and quality of life with the severely obese men and women having the lowest health domain scores (i.e., worst quality of life). With the exception of Mental Health, BMI had a graded inverse association with all SF-36 domains scores, with multivariate-adjusted scores lower for severely obese than for obese men and women who in turn had lower quality of life compared with normal weight or overweight individuals (p-values for

Table 1. Baseline Characteristics of 4,133 Men and 2,775 Women Ages 65+ in 2001 by Baseline BMI,[*] Chicago Heart Association Detection Project in Industry Study, 1967-73

	Baseline BMI (Kg/m^2)					
	Men			*Women*		
	18.5-<25.0	25.0-<30.0	≥30.0	18.5-<25.0	25.0-<30.0	≥30.0
Variable	n=1263	n=2339	n=531	n=1793	n=759	n=223
BMI	23.4 (1.3)	27.2 (1.4)	32.3 (2.5)[†]	22.2 (1.6)	26.9 (1.3)	33.6 (3.4)[†]
Age, years	42.1 (6.5)	42.7 (6.5)	43.0 (6.0)[†]	45.1 (6.6)	46.7 (6.6)	46.4 (6.8)[†]
Age at 2001, years	73.2 (6.3)	73.6 (6.3)	73.8 (6.0)	75.3 (6.5)	77.3 (6.6)	76.7 (6.8)[†]
African American race, %	2.1	2.8	3.6	5.5	7.9	8.1[†]
Blood pressure, mmHg						
Systolic	131.9 (14.8)	136.3 (15.5)	142.9 (17.3)[†]	128.0 (16.1)	134.2 (18.6)	143.2 (18.4)[†]
Diastolic	78.1 (9.6)	81.4 (9.9)	85.6 (10.9)[†]	76.3 (10.3)	79.6 (11.1)	84.1 (10.6)[†]
Serum cholesterol level, mg/dL	199.6 (33.8)	209.7 (36.7)	214.2 (35.4)[†]	206.0 (37.4)	211.3 (36.5)	216.9 (46.3)[†]
Current smoker, %	33.2	30.0	26.9[†]	32.0	23.1	22.0[†]
No. of cigarettes/d for smokers	22.3 (10.4)	22.2 (11.1)	23.8 (11.8)	17.7 (9.2)	15.7 (8.9)	16.6 (8.6)[†]
ECG abnormality						
Minor	4.9	5.2	7.3	3.1	5.1	5.8[†]
Major	4.2	3.8	4.3	8.8	8.6	7.6
Educational levels, years	14.3 (2.5)	14.0 (2.6)	13.6 (2.5)[†]	12.8 (2.2)	12.2 (2.2)	11.9 (2.1)[†]

*Body mass index, computed as weight in kilograms divided by square of height in meters.

†p<0.05 from F (continuous variables) or χ2 tests (categorical variables) of overall group differences.

Table 2. Definitions and Unadjusted Descriptive Statistics of Eight SF-36 Domains for Men and Women Ages 65+ in 2001

SF-36 Domain [*†]	Definition of Domain Score	Men (n=4,133)				Women (n=2,775)			
		Mean	SD[‡]	Median	IQR[§]	Mean	SD[‡]	Median	IQR[§]
Physical Functioning (10 items)	Overall self-perception of health	74.7	25.8	85.0	35.0	61.8	29.8	70.0	50.0
Role Limitations-Physical (4 items)	Degree of limitation in performing various physical activities	72.5	37.7	100.0	50.0	59.6	41.3	75.0	75.0
Bodily Pain (2 items)	Limitations on performance of work or regular activities due to physical health	74.0	22.4	74.0	38.0	65.3	25.2	72.0	43.0
General Health (5 items)	Degree of physical pain	69.6	19.6	72.0	25.0	67.0	21.0	72.0	30.0
Vitality (4 items)	Perceived level of energy	63.8	19.9	65.0	30.0	58.1	21.8	60.0	30.0
Social Functioning (2 items)	Degree of interference with social activities due to physical or emotional health	88.5	21.6	100.0	12.5	82.8	26.0	100.0	25.0
Role Limitations-Mental (3 items)	Limitations on work and daily activities due to emotional problems	88.8	26.3	100.0	0	81.2	33.6	100.0	33.3
Mental Health (5 items)	Feelings of nervousness or depression	81.8	14.5	84.0	16.0	77.9	16.8	80.0	24.0
Standardized Physical Component Score (PCS)		45.5	10.6	48.7	15.0	41.1	12.1	43.0	20.0
Standardized Mental Component Score (MCS)		55.1	7.6	57.2	7.3	53.9	9.4	56.7	64.6
Total Score [**]		100.6	13.9	104.6	17.1	95.1	16.1	98.7	24.2

*For each domain, categorical responses are scaled into numeric scores (ranging from 0-100) according to the SF-36 scoring protocol.
†Number of items comprising the domain.
‡Standard Deviation.
§Interquartile range.

Table 3. Adjusted[*] Mean Scores for Eight SF-36 questionnaire Domains and Mean Summary Score after 31-Years of Follow-Up According to 3 BMI categories at Baseline

	Baseline BMI (Kg/m^2)							
	Men				Women			
SF-36 Domains[†]	18.5-<25.0	25.0-<30.0	≥30.0	p-trend[‡]	18.5-<25.0	25.0-<30.0	≥30.0	p-trend[‡]
	n=1263	n=2339	n=531		n=1793	n=759	n=223	
Physical Functioning	79.2	74.3‖	65.5‖	<0.001	66.1‖	57.4‖	42.9‖	<0.001
Role Limitations-Physical	77.0	72.3‖	62.3‖	<0.001	63.7	55.2‖	42.3‖	<0.001
Bodily Pain	77.5	73.5‖	67.7‖	<0.001	68.2	62.6‖	51.6‖	<0.001
General health	71.6	69.7‖	64.3‖	<0.001	69.1	65.0‖	57.1‖	<0.001
Energy/Fatigue	65.5	63.8§	59.9‖	<0.001	60.1	55.9‖	49.6‖	<0.001
Social Functioning	90.4	88.3§	84.6‖	<0.001	84.6	80.9‖	74.5‖	<0.001
Role Limitations-Mental	90.0	89.1	84.7‖	<0.001	82.7	79.4¶	75.8§	<0.001
Mental Health	81.9	82.1	80.2¶	0.084	78.3	77.3	76.7	0.074
Standardized Physical Component Score (PCS)	47.4	45.3‖	41.6‖	<0.001	42.9	39.4‖	33.1‖	<0.001
Standardized Mental Component Score (MCS)	55.0	55.3	54.9	0.843	54.0	53.8	54.1	0.942
Total Score[**]	102.4	100.6‖	96.5‖	<0.001	96.8	93.2‖	87.2‖	<0.001

*Adjusted for age in 2001, race (indicator for black), education (years), smoking (cigarettes/day), any electrocardiographic abnormalities.

†For each domain, categorical responses are scaled into numeric scores (ranges 0-100) according to SF-36 scoring protocol.

‡p-values for linear trend across the three BMI categories.

§p<0.01, ‖p<0.001, ¶p<0.05 for comparisons with normal weight group (18.5-<25.0).

**Total score is computed as the sum of PCS and MCS.

trends were < 0.0001 for all). For example, multivariable-adjusted scores for General Health were 71.8, 69.7, 64.4, and 59.0, respectively for normal weight, overweight, obese, and severely obese men. Corresponding numbers for women were 69.1, 65.0, 58.4, and 53.4 (p-values for trend < 0.001). Similar relationships were obtained with the total score and PCS (i.e., for men, PCS scores were 47.4, 45.3, 42.1, and 36.6; and for women, PCS scores were 42.9, 39.4, 33.7, and 31.3 for those who were normal weight, overweight, obese, and severely obese, respectively) but not with the MCS score (p-values for trend < 0.001).

Age-adjusted prevalence of any reported difficulty in performing basic and instrumental activities of daily living (ADLs and IADLs) was also lower among men and women who were normal weight at baseline. Eighty-one percent of normal weight men and 79.6% of normal weight women reported no disability at follow-up, compared to 77.7% and 73.0% of overweight and obese men, and 73.5% and 62.5% of overweight and obese women (p-values < 0.001). Conversely, ADL disability or institutionalization (living in a nursing home) was reported by 2.9% of normal weight men compared to 3.2% of overweight and 7.0% of obese men; corresponding figures for women were 6.1%, 8.2%, 13.9% of women (p-values < 0.001). Similar trends were seen for prevalence of disability in IADLs only.

****

Since the beginning of the 20th century, there have been dramatic improvements in life expectancy, with decline in mortality before age 65 contributing substantially to these gains [Anderson RN, 1999]. An individual in the US reaching age 65 now can expect to live on average an additional 18 years, and life expectancy should continue to rise [Foot DK et al., 2000; National Center for Health Statistics 1999]. With the baby boomer generation poised to enter old age, it is estimated that by the year 2050, the population segment ages 65 years and older (currently comprising 12.4%) will grow to 20% of the US population, with the oldest old – that is, persons 85 years and older – comprising the fastest growing segment [Foot DK et al., 2000; National Center for Health Statistics 1999; US Census Bureau, 2001]. This trend in aging is a global phenomenon, with numbers of people ages 60 or older worldwide expected to increase from 1 in 10 currently, to 1 in 5 by 2050, and developing nations expected to face the greatest rate of population aging [United Nations Secretariat Dept of Economic and Social Affairs, 2003].

With more people surviving to older ages, it is becoming increasingly important to address not only morbidity, but also disability and poor quality of life that can accompany aging even in the absence of clinical disease. Some contend that increased life expectancy will lead to growing numbers of frail, disabled, and institutionalized older persons with decreased quality of life and increased costs for health care [Verbrugge LM, 1984; Crimmins EM et al., 1994; Schneider EL and Guralnik JM, 1990; Schneider EL and Brody JA, 1983; Spillman BC and Lubitz J, 2000]. Alternatively, as recently demonstrated, for the small percentage of persons (less than 10% of 39,573 CHA participants) with favorable baseline levels of all major CVD risk factors (i.e., at low risk) compared to all others, CHD/CVD is rare (endemic) not epidemic over the decades into older age; CHD/CVD death rates are remarkably low; death rates from cancers, other medical causes, and all-causes are considerably lower; longevity is greater by years; and average annual health care costs sizably lower [Stamler J et al., 1993; Stamler J et al., 1999; Daviglus ML et al., 1998].

Further more, low risk individuals have also been shown to have better self-reported health-related quality of life – a paramount issue among older people [Daviglus ML et al., 2003]. The ideal outcome of increased years of survival is to enjoy those years disability-free and healthy, a concept described by the compression of morbidity hypothesis, which proposes that while human life span has its limits, the age of onset of morbidity can be postponed, reducing the number of years spent with disability and disease to a brief period before death [Fries JF, 1980]. While this has not been conclusively proven, individuals with favorable health risk (determined by smoking status, BMI, and exercise patterns), experienced half the cumulative disability of those at high risk after 32 years of follow-up, and onset of disability was postponed by approximately 5 years in the low-risk compared to the high-risk group [Vita AJ et al., 1998]. Moreover, when the course of disability prior to death was examined among 418 decedents, those with fewer lifestyle risk factors experienced less overall disability, and accelerated decline of functional ability was delayed before death [Hubert HB et al., 2002]. These findings suggest that healthy habits and traits may lead to postponement of the onset of disability and lower lifetime disability.

Our main finding, based on an average follow-up of 31 years, is that BMI level in middle-aged men and women is significantly and independently related to various aspects of self-reported quality of life, i.e., physical, social, and mental well-being, in older age. Among normal weight individuals, preservation of health status was evident in the physical and social domains.

Scores for SF-36 domains measuring physical and social functioning as well as mental health were generally highest (best) in men and women with normal weight at baseline and decreased with higher BMI, with worst outcomes among severely obese individuals, although trends were not significant for mental health. A higher proportion of normal weight men and women had no limitation in common basic physical activities and perceived themselves as having excellent or very good health (important because poor subjective health has been shown to relate to mortality risk, independent of physical health) [Mossey JM and Shapiro MA, 1982; Kaplan GA and Camacho T, 1983; Pijls LTJ et al., 1993]. Both ADL and IADL disability were significantly more prevalent among overweight and obese men and women. The findings presented here – based on extended follow-up and widely used and well validated quality of life and disability instruments – are consistent with and confirm earlier results from the 26-year follow-up survey with quality of life assessed using the HSQ-12 questionnaire [Daviglus ML et al., 2003].

Much attention has been focused on the prevention of chronic diseases by prevention and control of major risk factors, with resultant reduction in mortality and increase in longevity. However, chronic disease risk factors, which can be largely asymptomatic, can also cause sub-clinical disease and affect quality of life [Daviglus ML et al., 2003; Chambers BA et al., 2002]. Overweight and obesity are important determinants of type 2 diabetes, insulin resistance, hypertension, and dyslipidemia [NHLBI Obesity Initiative Expert Panel, 1998] and are independently associated with future morbidity and mortality from CHD and CVD [Rimm EB et al., 1995; Calle EE et al., 1999; Dyer AR et al., 2004]. In addition, excess weight is strongly related to higher risk of some types of cancers (endometrial, prostate, colon, breast), gallbladder disease, osteoarthritis, sleep apnea, respiratory problems, and other conditions [Giovannucci E et al., 1996; Huang DJ et al., 1997; Stampfer MJ et al., 1992; Hart DJ and Spector TD, 1993]. Based on results of the CHA postal survey, which included a checklist of major diseases and conditions, normal weight individuals had significantly lower self-reported age-adjusted prevalence of any illness compared to those overweight and obese (i.e., 48.2% vs. 54.8%, and 65.3% respectively; p-values for trend < 0.001). Furthermore, high BMI levels have been shown to be associated with increased health care costs [Liu K et al., 1999; Quesenberry CP et al., 1998]. For example, among 9,046 men and 7,247 women from the CHA study, higher BMI in middle age (ages 33 – 64 at baseline in 1967-73) was significantly associated with higher multivariate-adjusted average annual and cumulative Medicare charges – total and for CVD-related care – in older age (1984-2000) [Daviglus ML et al., 2004].

Unlike most other coronary risk factors, prevalence of overweight and obesity are on the rise. Recent data from NHANES 1999-2000 show that age-adjusted prevalence of overweight and obesity among US adults are 34% and 31%, respectively, up from 33% and 23% in 1994 [Kuczmarski RJ et al., 1994; Flegal KM et al., 1998; Flegal KM et al., 2002]. Furthermore, although BMI is directly and independently associated with long-term CVD and total mortality [Dyer AR et al., 2004], the proportions of CHA participants surviving to at least age 65 ranged from 80% (severely obese) to 89% (non-overweight) for men and from 91% (severely obese) to 95% (non-overweight) for women [Daviglus ML et al., 2004]. Hence a large proportion of persons who are overweight and obese earlier in life will live to suffer its deleterious consequences in older age: more disease and disability, with accompanying higher health care costs. With the current trends of increasing BMI and the aging of the US population, implementation of preventive measures at younger ages is urgently required to lessen and contain future individual and societal burden of disease, health care costs, and disability and impaired quality of life associated with excess weight.

The determinants of obesity are complex and multifactorial, with genetic, biologic, behavioral, social, and environmental contributions. While genetic and biologic factors that predispose certain individuals and populations to weight gain have not yet been fully elucidated, it is certain that most if not all levels of susceptibility are intensified by adverse environmental factors – all too common in our modern society – that promote physical inactivity and over-consumption of food. Prevention and control of overweight and obesity is fraught with difficulties related to consumption of calorie-rich foods, sedentary lifestyles, and insufficient as well as ineffective treatment options. Weight control is a commonly reported behavior, and consumers spend more and more each year on weight loss programs and products. In a 1998 national telephone survey, 29% of men and 44% of women reported trying to lose weight, however, most were not following the recommended combination of reduced caloric intake and increased physical activity, which may explain ineffectiveness of most weight loss attempts [Serdula MK et al., 1999]. Moreover, although persons who are advised by their physicians to lose weight are significantly more likely to attempt to do so, less than half of obese adults report receiving such advice from their physicians [Sciamanna C et al., 2000]. The US Preventive Task Force recommends that clinicians screen for obesity during the office visit [US Preventive Task Force, 2002]. Obesity screening strategies that may be adopted in clinical practice include counseling about health risks of obesity, prescribing increased physical activity and weight loss, referral to nutritionists, and assisting patients in setting realistic and achievable goals [Manson JE et al., 2004].

Limitations of the CHA study include loss to follow-up for health assessment of a portion of eligible surviving original members of the CHA cohort, reflected in the response rate to the mailed survey (approximately 60%). Difficulties of long-term follow-up have been well documented, especially in studies where participants have not been contacted for decades, and response rates have been similar to ours [Clarke R et al., 1998]. As expected, in the CHA cohort, compared to non-responders of the follow-up survey, responders were younger, had more years of education, and were more likely to be men, white, and have a better CVD risk profile at baseline, i.e., lower mean blood pressure and serum total cholesterol levels and lower prevalence of diabetes and smoking. Additionally, response rate among participants determined to be obese at baseline has been found to be lower compared to those who were overweight and normal weight (54.7%, 60.6%, and 62.4%, respectively) [Daviglus ML et al., 2003]. This finding suggests that the associations between BMI and quality of life reported here are almost certainly underestimates, and that associations would have been stronger had we obtained a better response rate in the overweight and obese groups. A further limitation is that measurement of BMI was made at only a single point in time. Duration of overweight and obesity may well play an important role in lessening quality of life – a matter we could not assess. We also do not know how other factors related to obesity, such as physical inactivity or diet, may influence physical, mental, and social health. In addition, although participants with history of myocardial infarction or diagnosis of diabetes were excluded at baseline, it was not possible to exclude those who might have had cancer or other chronic diseases at initial examination, which might influence quality of life even decades later, because such information was not collected. Nevertheless, the likelihood is small that participants with cancer or other severe chronic diseases would still be surviving 31 or more years later. Moreover, the CHA cohort was derived from employed persons in Chicago; thus, they were likely to be healthier than the general population.

CONCLUSION

These results demonstrate that higher BMI in middle age adversely impacts future health-related quality of life and physical functioning in older age. Conversely, for non-overweight persons (BMI 18.5 – 24.9 kg/m^2), preservation of health status and quality of life is evident, indicating that increasing life expectancy can be accompanied with disease-free and disability-free survival. With a large segment of the US population now middle-aged and older facing trends of increasing obesity and overweight, preventive measures are urgently required to lessen future individual and societal burden of disease, disability, cost of care, and impaired quality of life associated with excess weight. By middle age, lifestyle patterns and risk factors, including excess weight, have often been established for decades. Moreover, successful long-term treatment of obesity is known to be difficult [Levy AS and Neaton AW, 1993; Eckel RH et al., 1998; Serdula MK et al., 1999; Kasirer JP and Angell M, 1998]. Thus, for those already overweight or obese, perhaps the only viable solution rests in the widespread deployment of innovative multi-faceted media and community based educational programs emphasizing the possibility of successful weight loss and weight maintenance through moderation of diet and increase in exercise. The decades-long national efforts against tobacco use that have resulted in a dramatic decline in adult smoking behavior may serve as models [National Cancer Institute, 1991]. However, as a long-term goal, we cannot limit ourselves only to a strategy emphasizing weight reduction and treatment of obesity. Instead, strategies that emphasize primary prevention of excess weight from an early age, with the potential of ending the obesity epidemic and leading to improved quality of life, should also become an ongoing component of national public health policy.

REFERENCES

American Heart Association. *Heart and Stroke Statistics – 2004 Update.* Dallas, Texas. American Heart Association, 2003.

Anderson RN, DeTurk PB. United States life tables, 1999. *National vital statistics reports*; Vol 50 no. 6. Hyattsville, Maryland. National Center for Health Statistics, 2002.

Apovian CM, Frey CM, Wood GC, Rogers JZ, Still CD, Jensen GL. Body mass index and physical function in older women. *Obesity Research.* 2002;10:740-7.

Calle EE, Thun MJ, Petrelli JM, Rodriguez C, Heath CW. Body mass index and mortality in a prospective cohort of US adults. *New Engl. J. Med.* 1999;341:1097-1105.

Chambers BA, Guo SS, Siervogel R, Hall G, Chumlea WMC. Cumulative effects of cardiovascular disease risk factors on quality of life. *J. Nutrition Health and Aging,* 2002;6:110-115.

Clarke R, Breeze E, Sherliker P, et al. Design, objectives, and lessons from a pilot 25 year follow up re-survey of survivors in the Whitehall study of London Civil Servants. *J. Epidemiol. Community Health* 1998;52:364-9.

Coakley EH, Kawachi I, Manson JE, Speizer FE, Willett WC, Colditz GA. Lower levels of physical functioning are associated with higher body weight among middle-aged and older women. *Int. J. Obes. Relat. Metab. Disord.* 1998;22:958-965.

Cooper R, Cutler J, Desvigne-Nickens P, et al. Trends and disparities in coronary heart disease, stroke, and other cardiovascular diseases in the United States. Findings of the National Conference on Cardiovascular Disease Prevention. *Circulation* 2000;102:3137-47.

Crimmins EM, Hayward MD, Saito Y. Changing mortality and morbidity rates and the health status and life expectancy of the older population. *Demography* 1994;31:159-75.

Daviglus ML, Liu K, Greenland P, Dyer AR, Garside DB, Manheim L, Lowe L, Rodin MB, Lubitz J, Stamler J. Benefits of a favorable cardiovascular risk-factor profile in middle age with respect to Medicare costs. *New Engl. J. Med.*1998; 339:1122-29.

Daviglus ML, Liu K, Pirzada A, Yan LL, Garside DB, Feinglass J, Guralnik JM, Greenland P, Stamler J. Favorable cardiovascular risk profile in middle age and health-related quality of life in older age. *Arch. Intern Med.* 2003;163:2460-8.

Daviglus ML, Liu K, Yan LL, Pirzada A, Garside DB, Schiffer L, Dyer AR, Greenland P, Stamler J. Body mass index in middle age and health-related quality of life in older age. The Chicago Heart Association Detection Project in Industry Study. *Arch. Intern Med.* 2003; 163:2448-2455.

Daviglus ML, Liu K, Yan LL, Pirzada A, Manheim L, Manning W, Garside DB, Wang R, Stamler J, Dyer AR, Greenland P. Relation of Body Mass Index in Middle Age to Medicare Expenditures in Older Age: The

Chicago Heart Association Detection Project in Industry [Manuscript submitted].

Doll HA, Petersen SEK, Stewart-Brown SL. Obesity and physical and emotional well-being: Associations between body mass index, chronic illness, and the physical and mental components of the SF-36 questionnaire. *Obesity Research* 2000;8:160-170.

Duke University Center for the Study of Aging and Human Development. Multidimensional functional assessment: the OARS methodology. 1978. Durham NC: Duke University.

Dyer AR, Stamler J, Garside DB, Greenland P. Long-term consequences of body mass index for cardiovascular mortality: The Chicago Heart Association detection Project in Industry Study. *Ann. Epidemiol.* 2004;14:101-108.

Eckel RH, Krauss RM for the American Heart Association Nutrition Committee. American Heart Association Call to Action: Obesity as a major risk factor for coronary heart disease. *Circulation* 1998;97:2099-2200.

Ferraro KF, Booth TL. Age, body mass index, and functional illness. *J. Gerontol. Soc. Sci.* 1999;54B:S339-348.

Ferraro KF, Su Y, Gretebeck RJ, Black DR, Badylak SF. Body mass index and disability in adulthood: A 20-year panel study. *Am. J. Public Health* 2002;92:834-840.

Flegal KM, Carroll MD, Kuczmarski RJ, Johnson CL. Overweight and obesity in the United States: prevalence and trends, 1960 – 1994. *Int. J. Obes.* 1998;22:39-47.

Flegal KM, Carroll MD, Ogden CL, Johnson CL. Prevalence and trends in obesity among US adults, 1999-2000. *JAMA* 2002;288:1723-27.

Foot DK, Lewis RP, Pearson TA, Beller GA. Demographics and cardiology, 1950 – 2050. *J. Am. Coll. Cardiol.* 2000;35:1067-81.

Ford ES, Moriarty DG, Zack MM, Mokdad AH, Chapman DP. Self-reported body mass index and health-related quality of life: findings from the Beavioral Risk Factor Surveillance System. *Obesity Research* 2001;9:21-31.

Fries JF. Aging, natural death, and the compression of morbidity. *New Engl. J. Med.* 1980;303:130-5.

Galanos AN, Pieper CF, Cornoni-Huntley JC, Bales CW, Fillenbaum GG. Nutrition and function: is there a relationship between body mass index and the functional capabilities of community-dwelling elderly? *J. Am. Geriatr. Soc.* 1994;42:368-373.

Giovannucci E, Colditz GA, Stampfer MJ, Willett WC. Physical activity, obesity, and risk of colorectal adenoma in women (United States). *Cancer Causes Control* 1996;7:253-263.

Han TS, Tijhuis MAR, Lean MEJ, Seidell JC. Quality of life in relation to overweight and body fat distribution. *Am. J. Public Health* 1998;88:1814-20.

Harris TB, Savage PJ, Tell GS, et al. Carrying the burden of cardiovascular risk in old age: associations of weight and weight change with prevalent cardiovascular disease, risk factors, and health status in the Cardiovascular Health Study. *Am. J. Clin. Nutr.* 1997;66:837-44.

Hart DJ, Spector TD. The relationship of obesity, fat distribution, and osteoarthritis in women in the general population: the Chingford Study. *J. Rheumatol.* 1993;20:331-335

Health Outcomes Institute. *Twelve-item health status questionnaire (HSQ-12) version 2.0 user guide.* Bloomington, MN: Health Outcomes Institute, 1996.

Huang DJ, Hankinson SE, Colditz GA, et al. Dual effects of weight and weight gain on breast cancer risk. *JAMA* 1997;278:1407-1411.

Hubert HB, Bloch DA, Oehlert JW, Fries JF. Lifestyle habits and compression of morbidity. *J. Gerontol. Ser. A Biol. Sci. Med. Sci.*2002; 57:M347-51.

Jenkins KR. Obesity's effects on the onset of functional impairment among older adults. *Gerontologist* 2004;44:206-16.

Kaplan GA, Camacho T. Perceived health and mortality: a nine year follow-up of the human population laboratory cohort. *Am. J. Epidemiol.* 1983;117:292-304.

Kasirer JP, Angell M. Losing weight – an ill-fated New Year's resolution. *N. Engl. J. Med.* 1998;338:52-4.

Katz DA, McHorney CA, Atkinson RL. Impact of obesity on health-related quality of life in patients with chronic illness. *J. Gen. Intern Med.* 2000;15:789-796.

Katz S, Akpom CA. Index of ADL. *Medical Care.* 1976;14(5 Suppl):116-8.

Katz S, Ford AB, Moskowitz RW, Jackson BA, Jaffe MW. The index of ADL: A standardized measure of biological and psychosocial function. *JAMA* 1963;185:9091-4.

Kuczmarski RJ, Flegal KM, Campbell SM, Johnson CL. Increasing prevalence of overweight among U.S. adults. *JAMA* 1994;272:205-11.

Launer LJ, Harris T, Rumpel C, Madans J. Body mass index, weight change, and risk of mobility disability in middle-aged and older women. *JAMA* 1994;271:1093-8.

Lean MEJ, Han TS, Seidell JC. Impairment of health and quality of life using new US federal guidelines for the identification of obesity. *Arch. Intern Med.* 1999;159:837-43.

Levine JB, Zak B. Automated determination of serum cholesterol. *Clin. Chim. Acta,* 1964;10:381-84.

Levy AS, Neaton AW. Weight control practices of U.S. adults trying to lose weight. *Ann. Intern Med.* 1993;119:661-6.

Liu K, Daviglus ML, Garside D, Greenland P, Lowe L, Dyer AR, Stamler J. Body mass index (BMI) in middle age and health care costs in older age: the Chicago Heart Association Detection Project in Industry (CHA) Study. [Abstract]. *Circulation* 1999;99:1104-25.

Lopez-Garcia E, Banegas Banegas JR, Gutierrez-Fisac JL, Perez-Regadera AG, Ganan LD, Rodriguez-Artalejo F. Relation between body weight and health-related quality of life among the elderly in Spain. *Int. J. Obes. Relat. Metab. Disord.* 2003;27:701-9.

Manson JE, Skerrett PJ, Greenland P, et al. The escalating pandemics of obesity and sedentary lifestyle. *Arch. Intern Med.* 2004;164:249-258.

Mossey JM, Shapiro MA. Self-rated health: a predictor of mortality among the elderly. *Am. J. Public Health.* 1982;72: 800-808.

National Cancer Institute. Strategies to control tobacco use in the United States. A blueprint for public health action in the 1990s. Smoking and tobacco control monograph 1. Bethesda MD: National Institutes of Health, National Cancer Institute, 1991. (NIH Publication No. 92-3316)

National Center for Health Statistics. *Health, United States, 1999. With Health and Aging Chartbook.* Hyattsville, Maryland: 1999.

NHLBI Obesity Education Initiative Expert Panel on the Identification, Evaluation, and Treatment of Overweight and Obesity in Adults. Clinical guidelines on the identification, evaluation, and treatment of overweight and obesity in adults. The Evidence Report. NIH Publication No. 98-4083, Bethesda MD, September 1998.

Ogden CL, Flegal KM, Carroll MD, et al. Prevalence and trends in overweight among US children and adolescents,1999-2000. *JAMA.* 2002;288:1728-1732.

Okoro CA, Hootman JM, Strine TW, Balluz LS, Mokdad AH. Disability, arthritis, and body weight among adults 45 years and older. *Obesity Research* 2004; 12:854-61.

Pijls LTJ, Feskens EJM, Kromhout D. Self-rated health, mortality and chronic diseases in elderly men. The Zutphen Study, 1985-1990. *Am. J. Epidemiol.* 1993;138:840-848.

Population Division, Department of Economic and Social Affairs, United Nations Secretariat. *The aging of the world's population.* January 2003. Available at: http://www.un.org/esa/socdev/ageing/agewpop.htm. Accessed June 20, 2004.

Prineas RJ, Castle CH, Curb JD, Harrist R, Lewin A, Stamler J. Hypertension detection and follow-up program: baseline electrocardiographic characteristics of the hypertensive participants. *Hypertension* 1983;5:IV160-IV189.

Priyanath A, Daviglus ML, Dyer AR, Liu K, Greenland P, Stamler J. Relationship of body mass index and coronary heart disease mortality in young adults. The Chicago Heart Association Detection Project in Industry. *Jap. J. Cardiovasc. Disease Prev.* 2001;36(Suppl):13.

Quesenberry CP, Caan B, Jacobson A. Obesity, health services use, and health care costs among members of a health maintenance organization. *Arch. Intern Med.* 1998;158:466-72.

Rimm EB, Stampfer MJ, Giovannucci E, Ascherio A, Spiegelman D, Colditz GA, Willett WC. Body size and fat distribution as predictors of CHD among middle aged and older US men. *Am. J. Epidemio.* 1995;141:1117-27.

Rosenbloom AL, Young RS, Joe JR, et al. Emerging epidemic of type 2 diabetes in youth. *Diabetes Care.* 1999;22:345-354.

Rosow I. Breslau N. A Guttman health scale for the aged. *J. Gerontol.* 1966;21:556-9.

Schneider EL, Brody JA. Aging, natural death and the compression of morbidity: another view. *New Engl. J. Med.* 1983;309:854-55.

Schneider EL, Guralnik JM. The aging of America: impact on health care costs. *JAMA* 1990;2335-2340.

Sciamanna CN, Tate DF, Lang W, et al. Who reports receiving advice to lose weight? Results from a multistate survey. *Arch. Intern Med.* 2000;160:2334-2339.

Serdula MK, Mokdad AH, Williamson DF, Galuska DA, Mendlein JM, Heath GW. Prevalence of attempting weight loss and strategies for controlling weight. *JAMA* 1999;282:1353-58.

Sinha R, Fisch G, Teague B, et al. Prevalence of impaired glucose tolerance among children and adolescents with marked obesity. *New Engl. J. Med.* 2002;346:802-10.

Spillman BC, Lubitz J. The effect of longevity on spending for acute and long-term care. *New Engl. J. Med.* 2000;342:1409-15.

Stamler J, Dyer AR, Shekelle RB, Neaton J, Stamler R. Relationship of baseline major risk factors to coronary and all-cause mortality, and to longevity: findings from long-term follow-up of Chicago cohorts. *Cardiology* 1993;82;191-222.

Stamler J, Rhomberg P, Schoenberger JA, Shekelle RB, Dyer A, Shekelle S, Stamler R, Wannamaker J. Multivariate analysis of the relationship of seven variables to blood pressure: findings of the Chicago Heart Association Detection Project in Industry, 1967-1972. *J. Chronic. Dis.* 1975;28:527-548.

Stamler J, Stamler R, Neaton JD, Wentworth D, Daviglus ML, Garside D, Dyer AR, Liu K, Greenland P. Low risk-factor profile and long-term cardiovascular and non-cardiovascular mortality and life expectancy. Findings for 5 large cohorts of young adult and middle-aged men and women. *JAMA* 1999;282:2012-2018.

Stampfer MJ, Maclure KM, Colditz GA, Manson JE, Willett WC. Risk of symptomatic gallstones in women with severe obesity. *Am. J. Clin. Nutr.* 1992;55:652-658.

Sternfeld B, Ngo L, Satariano WA, Tager IB. Associations of body composition with physical performance and self-reported functional limitation in elderly men and women. *Am.J. Epidemiol.* 2002;156:110-21.

The Pooling Project Research Group. Relationships of blood pressure, serum cholesterol, smoking habit, relative weight, and ECG abnormalities to incidence of major coronary events: Final Report of the Pooling Project. *J. Chron. Dis.* 1978;31:201-306.

Tibblin G, Svarsudd K, Welin L, Erikson H, Larsson B. Quality of life as an outcome variable and a risk factor for total mortality and cardiovascular disease: A study of men born in 1913. *J. Hyperten – Supplement.* 1993;11:S81-S86.

Troiano RP, Flegal KM. Overweight children and adolescents: description, epidemiology, and demographics. *Pediatrics.* 1998;101:497-504.

U.S. Census Bureau. Profiles of general demographic characteristics. 2000 Census of Population and Housing, United States. Issued May 2001. Available at: *http://www.census.gov/Press-Release/www/2001/demopr ofile.html.* Accessed: June 15, 2004.

US Preventive Services Task Force. Behavioral counseling in primary care to promote physical activity: recommendation and rationale. *Ann. Intern Med.* 2002;137:208-215.

Verbrugge LM. Longer life but worsening health? Trends in health and mortality of middle-aged and older persons. *Milbank Q* 1984;62:475-19.

Visscher TL, Rissanen A, Seidell JC, Heliovaara M, Knekt P, Reunanen A, Aromaa A. Obesity and unhealthy life-years in adult Finns. *Arch. Intern Med.* 2004;164:1413-1420.

Vita AJ, Terry RB, Hubert HB, Fries JF. Aging, health risks, and cumulative disability. *New Engl. J. Med.* 1998;338:1035-41.

Walters SJ, Munro JF, Brazier JE. Using the SF-36 with older adults: a cross-sectional community-based survey. *Age Ageing.* 2001;30:337-43.

Ware JE Jr, Snow KK, Kosinski M, Gabdek B. *SF-36 Health Survey: Manual and Interpretation Guide.* Boston, Mass: The Health Institute, New England Medical Center; 1993.

Ware JE, Kosinski M, Bayliss MS, McHorney CA, Rogers WH, Raczek A. Comparison of methods for the scoring and statistical analysis of SF-36 health profile and summary measures: summary of results from the Medical Outcomes Study. *Medical Care.* 1995;33:AS264-279.

Wolf AM, Colditz GA. Current estimates on the economic cost of obesity in the United States. *Obesity Research* 1998;6:97-100.

Yan LL, Daviglus ML, Liu K, Pirzada A, Garside DB, Schiffer L, Dyer AR, Greenland P. BMI and health-related quality of life in adults 65 years and older. *Obesity Research.* 2001;12:69-76.

Yancy WS, Olsen MK, Westman EC, Bosworth HB, Edelman D. Relationship between obesity and health-related quality of life in men. *Obesity Research* 2002;10:1057-64.

INDEX

D

E

L

M

N

Q

R

T

U

V